DIABETES

DIABETES

The Psychology of Control

Val Wilson

<teneo> //press
AMHERST, NEW YORK

Requests for permission should be directed to
webmaster@teneopress.com, or mailed to:
Teneo Press
c/o Cambria Press
100 Corporate Parkway, Suite 128
Amherst, New York 14226, USA

ISBN: 978-1-934844-53-3

For Neil

TABLE OF CONTENTS

DIABETES

INTRODUCTION

Diabetes occurs when there is a change in the way the body can use glucose, causing there to be an increase of glucose in the blood due to a lack of insulin to correct this imbalance. In Type 1 diabetes, insulin is no longer produced and in Type 2, there is increased insulin production which cannot be used effectively. Diabetes is now a huge challenge for health services in terms of provision and cost as numbers with the condition have escalated to epidemic proportions in recent years. Type 2 diabetes, which accounts for 90 percent of all cases, occurs in the majority of patients due to poor diet and a sedentary lifestyle, representing the alarming worldwide increase in diabetes in the 21st century.

Because diabetes can lead to a number of serious complications, such as eye and kidney disease and heart and circulatory system disorders, the patient must learn to manage their condition so that blood glucose levels are kept within the range of a non-diabetic individual to minimise this risk. This means that unlike any other chronic health condition, people with diabetes deliver more than 95 percent of their own care. Unsurprisingly this demand takes a considerable toll on the physical and psychological wellbeing of the patient, both in terms of the initial diagnosis of the disease, and regarding the ongoing long-term challenges faced by those who have had diabetes for many years.

Whilst living well with diabetes requires a good level of care by both health professionals and the patient, the physical consequences of diabetes are deeply interwoven with the psychological health of the individual. These consequences may be perceived as negligible or devastating depending on issues such as the degree of disability and the level of disruption to the person's life, the individual's coping style, the presence of other competing health conditions that must also be managed, and the individual's perceptions of the health challenges they face. Recognising why and how these issues impact the self-management of diabetes is the first step towards being able to address these problems.

ABOUT THIS BOOK

Dr Val Wilson is a specialist in diabetes health education, having spent eighteen years involved in diabetes research, including over ten years of voluntary work with the INPUT (Insulin Pump Therapy) national diabetes organisation. Dr Wilson has conducted numerous independent studies concerning how people self-manage their diabetes, and this book contains anonymous quotes from people with the condition to illustrate the patient's perspective of the issues highlighted in each chapter.

As an individual with long-duration Type 1 diabetes that is difficult to manage, Dr Wilson offers the insight of a person living with the condition to *Diabetes: The Psychology of Control.* It aims to cover the multitude of psychosocial issues that affect people with diabetes on a day-to-day basis, with the understanding that it is not just as simple as following the advice of health professionals in order to manage the condition effectively. This book begins by exploring the perspective of health professionals and the theories behind how diabetes care is offered to the patient, including examples of the individual's perspective of the care they receive and how they manage their diabetes according to their circumstances. The burden of depression, for example, means that diabetes is more difficult to self-manage as depression leads to increased blood glucose levels and often a reduction in the individual's ability to carry out self-care activities.

The brain is continually influenced by chemical processes that have a significant impact on how diabetes is managed in terms of thoughts, decisions and subsequent health-related behaviour. Emotions also play an important central role in consciousness and awareness that influence thoughts and activities which are expressed in decision making and behaviour. Behaviour and emotions can be altered by the individual using techniques that increase awareness of potentially poor health behaviours. In time, this can lead to a number of health benefits as changes occur in the way the person thinks and reacts to challenges such as pain and depression. It may not be possible for a person with very difficult to control Type 1 diabetes to manage their condition well. This is made an even greater challenge if they also adopt disordered eating behaviour in an attempt to lose weight, maintain weight loss, or as a control mechanism in order to cope with stressful life events.

Type 1 diabetes is a condition where the immune system, which usually fights infection, attacks its own insulin-producing cells and produces antibodies that continue to destroy these cells for the rest of the person's life. Because of this fault in the immune system it is common that other auto-immune conditions, such as asthma, coeliac disease, or thyroid disorders, also occur in the same person. This means that the individual has to manage multiple chronic health conditions, often presenting increasing problems with diabetes control. Because Type 2 diabetes is at epidemic proportions much research has focussed on reversing the condition, which is increasingly possible with surgical weight loss, enabling insulin to function normally in the body once more. However, weight loss surgery is not a quick fix and it is often accompanied by a number of psychological issues that must be addressed.

CHAPTER 1

DIABETES DENIAL

Diabetes is a complex metabolic disease that requires the patient to diligently self-manage blood glucose and other factors, such as cholesterol levels, at all times. These demands may lead to non-concordance with medical advice because of the overwhelming impact diabetes and its complications has on the individual psychologically and socially. For this reason, the diabetes care provided by health professionals needs to recognise the psychosocial factors that shape how and why individuals chose to care for their condition. From diagnosis, the individual's health beliefs, health goals and motivations shape their diabetes self-care and self-management behaviour, and this may change as duration of the condition increases.

The importance of psychosocial issues having an impact on people with diabetes has become more prominent since the publication of the National Service Framework (NSF) for Diabetes: Standards document (Department of Health, 2003a). NSF Standard 3 highlights the need for people with the condition to receive structured health education in addition to psychological support to assist with their self-management. The aim of this standard is to enable people to engage in self-care of their diabetes to the best extent achievable. The need for patient-centred psychological care for those with diabetes has been suggested by other researchers (Barry and Edgman, 2012; Lucas and Walker, 2004; Pouwer, et al., 2001), although Wilson (2003a) conducted a survey showing that 92.0 percent of 155 people with diabetes did not have a psychologist or trained counsellor as part of their diabetes team. Although it has been reported that 10 percent (£869 million annually) of the NHS budget goes on treating diabetes in the UK (BBC, 2015a) this accounts for medication and surgical procedures rather than providing counselling. The issue of sparse psychological support for people with diabetes is therefore set to continue as NHS funding in the United Kingdom is stretched to capacity.

Obesity carries with it risk of developing Type 2 diabetes which is 80 times greater than for the non-obese (McPherson, et al., 2007), with the number of people becoming obese and going on to develop Type 2 continuing to rise steadily in both adults and children due to lifestyle factors (Wanless, et al., 2007; Butless, et al., 2007). A diagnosis of diabetes brings with it not only physical consequences, but it also has a psychological impact affecting the individual and everyone around them (Clark, 2004). These factors include coping with the initial diagnosis; awareness of the potential secondary health conditions that accompany diabetes if it is not well-controlled, such as blindness, kidney failure, amputation, stroke, and heart disease; the cognitive effects (the process of gaining knowledge about diabetes, including perceptions and reasoning); and the psychological factors influenced by the condition, such as depression. The following comments from patients describe how a diagnosis of diabetes impacted on them:

> I was frightened to death by the mention of blindness because my grandmother had Type 2 diabetes, and that's what happened to her.

> I bought a couple of books about diabetes when I developed Type 1 as an adult. The photographs of amputated limbs and huge leg ulcers were difficult to take in – I thought that it couldn't happen to me.

I've had Type 1 for nearly 40 years and I've noticed that now I'm less keen to go out in case I have a low blood sugar attack. I also get very depressed and have been told [by a clinical psychologist] that I just have to accept it as it goes with the diabetes. It seems as though diabetes has taken over my whole life and I hate it.

The Department of Health National Service Framework for Diabetes (Department of Health, 2003b) states that diabetes self-management is the key to good diabetes care. The document suggests that 'good' diabetes self-management can be achieved by the individual with the provision of information, education and psychological support from their diabetes health professionals:

> People with diabetes need the knowledge, skills and motivation to assess their risks, to understand what they will gain from changing their behaviour or lifestyle, and to act on that understanding by engaging in appropriate behaviours.

Over the past 30 years the psychological effects of diabetes have been identified and characterised. Studies show that the impact of diabetes on the individual's mental health increases in accordance with the length of time that individual has had diabetes because the burden of the condition and its complications becomes greater (Anderson, et al., 2001; Ledhill, et al., 2000). Burns (2001) stated that when an individual becomes disabled due to a physical condition or an accident, their concept of self becomes damaged so that they ask questions like, 'Why me?'; they are forced to assess the extent to which their disability interferes with their normal life; and they begin to construct new approaches to a new set of activities, attitudes and social relationships. These issues are dealt with by trying to reduce the impact of the disability and the use of technical assistance, although Burns (2001) suggested that it is not sufficient to advise the individual learns to cope with physical or psychological problem by adjusting to their circumstances and accepting change.

THEORIES OF BEHAVIOUR APPLIED TO DIABETES

There has been a great amount of theoretical work attempting to explain human behaviour in terms of how people act when they are told they have a chronic health condition, and how they go on to manage that condition. Type 1 diabetes requires the individual, often a child, to adopt a diligent self-management regime including multiple daily insulin injections, or insulin pump therapy (also known as Continuous Subcutaneous Insulin Infusion – CSII), regular self-monitoring of blood glucose levels throughout the day and often during the night as well, and continual monitoring of diet and exercise. This level of self-care, which is constantly required and unlike any other chronic health condition, is carried out in order to achieve near normal blood glucose levels of between 4.0–7.0 mmol/L (or 72–126mg/dl US measurement).

However, in some cases, Type 1 diabetes is very difficult to self-manage because good glycaemic (blood glucose) control cannot be easily achieved and this is termed 'brittle' diabetes. An individual may therefore do everything they can to manage their Type 1 to the best of their abilities, but may still fail to achieve this. This lack of control over the condition can lead to the person giving up trying to achieve near-normal blood glucose levels, or conversely they may become over-diligent in their attempts to attain control:

> My [Type 1] diabetes has always been really difficult to deal with so I inject twice a day and then forget about it. I figure that there is nothing I can do that will make any difference.

> Although I have very volatile [Type 1] diabetes, I try very hard to manage it with insulin pump therapy and blood testing six times a day, and I get on my exercise bike for half an hour after evening meals so I don't get a sharp rise in blood glucose.

In order to determine why some individuals are not positively engaged in their diabetes self-management, many of the approaches adopted in diabetes health education research and practice are rooted in the social and behavioural sciences, especially psychology. It has been argued that psychological theories are very relevant to diabetes education because they attempt to explain the individual's health behaviour and the way that person adapts to any change (Dixon, 2008; Peyrot and Rubin, 2007; Wilson, 2007). As a result, attempts have been made to unify different theories of health behaviour, which often have similar concepts (Noar and Zimmerman, 2005; Michie, et al., 2005), although this has proved impossible as the reasons why an individual is motivated to make changes to, or maintain their health behaviour are numerous and complex. Michie and colleagues (2005) have identified 12 different factors that affect motivation, including knowledge; skills; the individual's social and professional role and identity; the individual's perceived capabilities; beliefs about the consequences of an action; motivation and goals; memory; the individual's attention to the decision process; the environmental context and resources; social influences; emotion; behavioural regulation; and the nature of the behaviour.

Theories often propose models – an example or pattern that people may wish to follow. Two of the most prominent theories of behaviour that have been used in diabetes clinical practice are the Health Belief model [HBM] (Becker and Janz, 1985; Janz and Becker, 1984; Becker, 1974) and the Stages of Change model [SoC] (Prochaska and DiClemente, 1984). The HBM, when applied to diabetes, describes the individual's progression through a series of stages towards a positive behavioural change in their diabetes self-management. There are a number of other models which have developed from the HBM, such as Social Learning Theory [SLT] which has been used to describe the way individuals with the condition perceive the benefits of diabetes self-management behaviour, and their own role in terms of 'self-efficacy' (Kaplan, 1985; Bandura, 1977a). The Theory of Reasoned Action [TRA] has also developed from the HBM to describe the beliefs the individual has in the outcome of a certain behaviour and the value they attach to these outcomes (Azjen and Fishbein, 1975).

Diabetes and Social Learning Theory

Social Learning Theory concerns the two constructs of self-efficacy – the confidence the individual has to self-manage their diabetes effectively by normalising blood glucose levels to reduce the risk of diabetic complications; and outcome expectancy – the expected result of this diabetes self-management behaviour. The first of these constructs has become more prominent in diabetes care. SLT suggests that, in order for a particular behaviour to occur, the individual must have the expectation of a reward or outcome for that behaviour. Bandura (1977a) argued that whether a person continues with a particular behaviour when they alter their circumstances, for example, going on holiday and maintaining regular blood glucose testing, depends on their perception of their mastery over that behaviour. This can be seen in the following comments from people with diabetes:

> I always do plenty of blood glucose tests when I'm on holiday to make sure I'm on track as I don't want it spoilt by becoming ill.

> When we were moving house last year it was very stressful and difficult to maintain regular blood glucose testing, but I managed it because it is so important.

Bandura (1977b) felt that this sense of 'self-efficacy' developed through the individual's personal experiences of success, and also from verbal support from others. A study by Kaplan (1985) showed that the driving force behind the individual's intention to effectively undertake diabetes management behaviour was their outcome expectancy and their expectation that these self-care behaviours would improve glycaemic control. Other researchers have also found that perceived self-efficacy predicts participation in physical activity (Robbins, et al., 2004; McAuley and Blissmer, 2000; Broman, 1995). However, this has been questioned because exercise increases the levels of 'feel-good' endorphins in the brain, meaning any results may not be due to self-efficacy alone. In terms of managing diabetes though, self-efficacy seems to explain, to some degree, why the individual feels able to achieve and maintain good glycaemic control, especially if health professionals encourage diabetes self-management efforts.

A number of health-related studies have shown that the concept of self-efficacy can be put into practice to act as a coping strategy in chronic illness (Schwarzer and Fuchs, 1995). Taylor, et al. (1995) found that the recovery of cardiovascular functioning in patients who had suffered a heart attack was enhanced by the perception of their own coping ability. Arthritis sufferers using a cognitive behavioural therapy programme [which can help overcome destructive behavioural patterns] experienced a greater perception that they could manage their condition, having less pain and joint inflammation as a result (O'Leary, et al., 1988). Kaplan, et al. (1984) found that patients with chronic obstructive pulmonary diseases who had followed a self-efficacy training programme were better able to stick to their medical regime (concordance).

It could be argued that individuals with diabetes need coping strategies to help them manage the day-to-day demands of their condition. The evidence from studies examining self-efficacy in other chronic health conditions shows that if the individual feels they can manage their condition well their health is markedly improved. Self-efficacy has been described as a health belief by Tones and Tilford (1994). For people who have achieved good control of their diabetes, the individual's ability in their belief to manage their condition effectively, and their belief that carrying out self-care activities will have a specific outcome on their diabetes, suggests that the individual has consciously made a decision about their health-related behaviour. However, some people may avoid those diabetes self-care activities that they believe exceed their coping abilities, as can be seen in the following comments:

> When I'm feeling down, I eat what I like although I know I shouldn't as I have no way [with Type 2 diabetes, not on insulin] to bring down my high blood glucose.

> I find regular blood testing very difficult and inconvenient – trying to remember to do it and because it often hurts.

The concepts of control of a chronic disease, and the idea of empowerment (increasing the individual's understanding and potential for diabetes self-care), are closely linked to self-efficacy and are often applied to the management of diabetes. For this reason, other models such as the Diabetes Empowerment Scale have been developed to measure diabetes self-management behaviour (Anderson, et al., 2000). This study showed that diabetes education delivered by health professionals had to address issues that the patient wanted to tackle in order for self-efficacy to develop. Therefore, the concepts of self-efficacy and patient empowerment are strongly related to the diabetes care delivered by health professionals.

The principle of self-efficacy implies that individuals with poor self-efficacy are more likely to carry out harmful health-related behaviours, such as not testing blood glucose regularly. In terms of diabetes education, self-efficacy has additional benefits for health professionals who are trying to help their patients. Tones and Tilford (1994) have suggested that self-efficacy enables the application of practical techniques for enhancement of the patient's health beliefs. With this in mind, health professionals then aim to increase the individual's sense of self-efficacy in their own diabetes care, accompanied by structured and ongoing diabetes education (Department of Health, 2005).

Diabetes and the Health Belief Model

The Health Belief Model is used by diabetes health professionals because it suggests that health behaviour is based on how the individual appraises their susceptibility to a disease and its complications, and that their belief that taking preventable action will be effective in reducing this susceptibility (Becker, 1974). The individual's perception of a health risk is dependent on their weighing up the pros and cons that might result from adopting a particular health behaviour. Risk perception is therefore key to the role of certain health beliefs in stimulating preventable health actions. Not only must the individual believe that they are susceptible to a disease and its consequences, they must also perceive that it is serious in order to bring about consideration of preventative behaviour. A belief that this behaviour will be effective, and that the benefits outweigh the cost or disadvantages, must also be in place (Tones and Tilford, 1994). It could be assumed that individuals with diabetes perceive that they must manage their disease effectively in order to prevent chronic complications. However, this is not always the case (Diabetes UK, 2006). This suggests that many people with diabetes have difficulty in accepting the condition, and the constant demands it places on them, as demonstrated by the following comments:

> It's not really serious – it's only Type 2.

> I get told by the nurse that I should test my blood glucose levels before I drive, but I forget and it's too much hassle.

Disincentives for individuals to improve their health behaviour were classified into four categories thirty years ago by Dishman (1986) as effort, time, health limitations, and obstacles. This research concluded that these 'barriers' were likely to be the individual's own excuses for not changing behaviour rather than explanations for it. The HBM also described four common reasons for not changing health behaviour: perceived susceptibility to the condition; the perceived severity of the condition; perceived benefits of change; and perceived barriers to change. Further factors have been added to recognise self-efficacy: the individual must believe that they are capable of adopting a change in health behaviour. The individual may therefore reason that they cannot diligently manage their diabetes well all of the time because of the necessary time and effort this takes, as well as the individual's perception of chronic complications if no symptoms are present. Even if complications are present, the individual may be unable to effectively self-manage very difficult to control (brittle) Type 1 diabetes, shown by the following views:

> Despite having the necessary knowledge and available technology [insulin pump therapy], because my diabetes control is virtually unmanageable, I have retinopathy [diabetic eye disease] and severe neuropathy [nerve damage].

> I think the complications of diabetes will occur anyway over time because you can't keep blood sugar under control all the time.

Although various reasons have been found to predict numerous health behaviours and outcomes, there has been less attempt to change outcomes by changing how people think about their condition (Broome and Llewelyn, 1995). The motivating factor, or belief, represents the influences of social pressures on behaviour, such as conforming to peer group ideals (Dixon, 2008; Katz and Peberdy, 2001). This situation may lead to poor health behaviour, such as the young adolescent with Type 1 diabetes who consumes excess alcohol, despite its adverse effect of causing marked glucose fluctuations (Emanuele, et al., 1998). This high-lights a deficiency in the Health Belief Model in that it assumes that the individual evaluates the cost and benefit before considering a change in health behaviour, and the model fails to take account of influences such as family and friends, as well as assuming a high degree of rationality on behalf of the individual (Naidoo and Wills, 1994). Because the individual's healthcare behaviour is shaped by so many influences, it is difficult to fully describe why some individuals are concordant and achieve very diligent diabetes self-management whilst others do not.

As we have seen, several studies in the context of diabetes regime concordance have used the theoretical framework of the HBM, but this model has failed to provide a full explanation of diabetes self-management behaviour. According to the HBM, the individual's personal beliefs about their diabetes regime should be reflected in the self-care behaviours actually performed. However, it has been suggested that the findings for diabetes studies applying concepts of the HBM are inconsistent and contradictory, and that this is the case for all age groups (Shilitoe,

1988). Broome and Llewelyn (1995) have also stated that researchers have used different versions of the HBM in order to predict diabetes regime concordance, many of which have employed invalid measures and participants. It appears that the HBM can only be used to gain a certain amount of insight into diabetes management behaviour, but not the full picture of why and how people feel able to manage or not manage their diabetes correctly.

The HBM was originally used to predict 'compliance' with medical advice, such as taking up the offer of inoculations, so it does not fit with current diabetes care provision in that the model is not patient-centred. It is clear that being motivated to attend an appointment to receive an inoculation is very different to the commitment of managing a life-long chronic condition. In addition, the HBM fails to account for the influence of role models on the individual's decisions which affect their behaviour, and it assumes that the individual is always able to make rational decisions after weighing up all pros and cons before taking action. Because the HBM does not provide a full explanation of the concepts that are involved in altering or maintaining diabetes self-care behaviours, a patient-centred approach such as the Stages of Change model, is required.

Diabetes and the Stages of Change Model
It has often been stated that it is very difficult to encourage change in the self-care and self-management behaviours of people with diabetes, and that patients do not respond to advice. The Stages of Change (SoC) model, developed by Prochaska and DiClemente (1984) proposed a model of behaviour acquisition, which is important in showing that any change in behaviour does not end and is, in fact, a continual process. Although this model has been predominantly used to encourage change in addictive behaviours such as smoking and alcoholism (Prochaska, 1992; West, 2005), the SoC model is different to the HBM in that it acknowledges that the individual's decision-making occurs through five stages of willingness to change:

- Pre-contemplation
- Contemplation
- Planning or preparation
- Action
- Maintenance

At the pre-contemplation stage, the individual has not considered changing their lifestyle, or become aware of any potential risks to their health behaviour – for example, any symptoms of chronic complications or awareness of diabetes education in this respect. The contemplation stage is characterised by the individual's awareness of the benefits of change, and they may be seeking information or advice to help them make a decision. Therefore, a diabetes education message about chronic complications may then trigger the individual's risk perception. In the third stage, the individual views a change in behaviour as both possible and worthwhile and they are ready for the change to happen. Therefore, the individual becomes aware of the benefits of good control of diabetes to prevent or delay chronic complications and wants to gain information and support to help them adopt improved glycaemic control into their lifestyle.

The action stage involves a period of sustained decision-making to do things differently, with a clear goal, a realistic plan, and support. This is a much shorter stage: when commitment has been made, the individual moves to the final stage in the change process. Finally, the maintenance stage refers to sustained change, usually for longer than six months. The new behaviour is strengthened and develops into self-efficacy: thus the individual's feeling of being in control of their diabetes is maximised. Individuals progress through these stages in a cyclical way, rather than a linear fashion. Wilson (2009) has suggested that individuals do not always follow one stage after another, although they do go through all stages. Thus a relapse is not viewed as a failure, as the individual can go backwards as well as forwards.

The SoC model developed from a review of over 300 theories of mental health and illness and led to the identification of ten distinct processes of change underlying these theories (Marks, et al., 2000). Subsequent research has provided more detail about the various stages, and the process that connects them. The most important concepts of the SoC model are:

- The process of change
- Stages of change
- Decisional balance
- Self-efficacy
- Temptation

Janis and Mann (1977), in their decision-making model, proposed that two of these components, decisional balance and self-efficacy, enable the individual to move from one stage to another to help change to occur. Decisional balance – or weighing up the pros and cons of changing health behaviour – is a concept derived from the Health Belief Model. Self-efficacy – or the confidence the individual has to maintain behaviour change – is a concept of Bandura's (1977b) Social Learning Theory. The concepts of decisional balance and self-efficacy therefore assume that the individual is ready to change and improve their diabetes care behaviour having assessed the benefits, and that they are positive they can carry out and maintain the change they want to achieve.

Katz and Peberdy (1995) argue that behaviour is firmly rooted in the individual's psychological make-up and is located in social and cultural environments. Therefore, attempting to change behaviour in the name of health is an ethical issue, especially if the circumstances of the individual's life makes things difficult. For example, when applying this to diabetes self-management, the individual may be suffering from depression, making it difficult for them to perceive the benefits of a diabetes education message which is designed to help them attain an improved quality of life.

As we have seen, the SoC model focusses on the process of change and the support people might need. Webb and Sheeran (2006) have argued that attitudes are difficult to change, but that theoretically, changing one of three components will affect attitude: the cognitive; the effective; and the behavioural. The cognitive component is made up of the person's knowledge and information, and is the belief aspect (religion, culture, class, family background, peer group, and educational influences). The affective component of attitudes is concerned with emotions, feelings and preferences, and the behavioural aspect is determined by what people actually can do (the skills they have and the circumstances with which they have to contend). Thus, communicating a diabetes education message which counters a person's misinformed beliefs, for example, that diabetic eyes screening is only of benefit once retinopathy has begun to progress, may change the attitude of the individual so that they regard regular eye screening as a preventative measure for retinopathy.

Whilst individuals may not have an awareness of contemplating, actioning and maintaining behaviour change, the intention will be based upon the individual's decision that change is in their best interest (Naidoo and Wills, 1994). Thus, a successful diabetes education intervention will place emphasis on motivating the individual towards improved diabetes self-management. Taking smoking cessation as an example, evidence shows that individuals are more likely to be motivated to change their health-related behaviour if they are strongly involved in the planning process (MacLeod, et al., 1993). In terms of diabetes, it is clear that for effective self-management behaviour to take place, diabetes care must be patient-centred in recognising their needs.

The SoC model has rarely been used in its fullest form to help people with diabetes change behaviour but when it has been used, it has been with individuals who have Type 2 diabetes to help them focus on weight reduction in the United States (Ruggiero, 2000; Rossi, et al., 1997; Ruggiero and Prochaska, 1993). As this is the case it could be argued that the SoC model has only been used to change addictive behaviours because obesity can be described as an addiction to food. Since the application of the SoC model to Type 2 diabetes care in the United States, work has progressed from theory to practice. Ongoing research has focussed on large-scale clinical trials examining the impact of both stage-matched and individually-focussed interventions targeting multiple health behaviours in people with diabetes in the United States. Previous research looking at how individuals could successfully adopt and maintain Type 2 diabetes management behaviours has proved successful (Rossi, et al., 1997; 1994a; 1994b). This suggests that a patient-centred approach is useful for health professionals to adopt in the UK when delivering diabetes health education.

Criticisms have also been raised over the SoC model however in that there is little consistent evidence that this approach works. Bandura (1997) argued that the five stages of change were artificial, whilst Heather and Robertson (1997) suggested that behaviour change was often far more fluctuating than the model suggests. Although the SoC model is patient-centred, the individual may not be able to continually maintain good diabetes management behaviours once they have reached this stage and may return to the pre-contemplation stage if they, for example, experienced visual loss and were unable to carry out the same self-care activities. Losing a partner for a person with frequent and severe hypoglycaemia would also mean that they were unable to look after themselves if they require a glucagon injection when unconscious. These examples highlight that the SoC model describes the individual's perceptions at one particular stage, but not the effects of external issues which may cause relapse to an earlier stage, meaning that change is constantly fluctuating.

Prochaska and Velicier (1997a) responded that the stages are not a substitute for the process, but rather an attempt to identify when and where these processes operate. Prochaska and Velicier (1997b) also argued that the stage effect has been replicated in over 60 studies and has only failed in around six health conditions. Despite these criticisms the SoC model still provides a useful understanding of the individual's perspective concerning changing their behaviour within their current health and psychosocial status, although it does not tell us how or why a person moves from one stage to another.

PSYCHOSOCIAL ISSUES FOR PEOPLE WITH DIABETES

Adherence

Adherence is now termed concordance, referring to the extent that the individual follows a given medical treatment regime. The term 'non-concordance' is used to describe individuals who fail to follow the advice of health professionals. This can be thought of as a kind of reasoned decision-making, rather than a term implying that if health recommendations are not followed by the individual, they should be blamed. There is a school of thought which states that the altered metabolic parameters in diabetes mean that it is difficult, if not practically impossible, to rectify this imbalance, even if the person with diabetes is able to attain perfect control of their condition at all times. Although patient empowerment (informed choice) supports concordance and does not associate non-concordance with a diabetes self-management, the individual may make a decision not to concur with their advised treatment. This view has been described as rational decision-making by Day (1995), who stated that patients may chose to ignore a medical regime because they believe that their quality of life will be improved by doing so. Individuals with diabetes are therefore faced with a number of behavioural choices including concordance which involves numerous factors, from acting on the individual's own health beliefs, to the simple refusal to manage a complex and chronic medical condition (Donnovan, et al., 2002; Horne, 1997).

Concordance with a diabetes regime or health advice is difficult to measure because it often relies on the measurement of self-reported behaviour. What can be determined is the extent to which the individual engages in the behaviour they are reporting (Pouwer, et al., 2001). The frequency of prescription requests for blood glucose test strips, and the results of HbA1c blood glucose measurements (the amount of glucose sticking to the red blood cells over a 3-month period) can be correlated with the self-management behaviour the individual is reporting to health professionals. It is also known that certain health behaviours, such as following dietary recommendations, monitoring glucose levels, taking exercise regularly, and taking the correct amount of medication at the right time, are not strongly related to one another. This suggests that some aspects of diabetes self-management are more likely to be undertaken than others. This is common for all health behaviours where, for example, Ley (1992) found that almost 50 percent of patients forgot to take prescribed antibiotic medication.

Concordance is a behaviour that does not remain the same over time and it has been shown to increase in accordance with the length of time the individual has had diabetes (Chatterjee, 2006; Kovacs, et al., 1990). Connor and Norman (1996) have suggested that some inappropriate health behaviours are sustained because the individual with diabetes receives a lack of support for changing that behaviour. Non-concordance is a major barrier to the use of diabetes treatments such as multiple daily insulin injections or insulin pump therapy because they require diligence and motivation to use them effectively. These methods are often the only way to achieve optimum diabetes self-management, but these treatments involve the adoption of an intensive diabetes regime and for the individual to be proactive in their diabetes care. They must want and be enabled to improve their glycaemic control to prevent or delay the chronic complications of diabetes, such as eye and kidney disease.

Both the Diabetes Control and Complications Trial (DCCT, 1993) for Type 1 diabetes, and the UK Prospective Diabetes Study (UKPDS, 1998a, UKPDS, 1998b) for Type 2 diabetes, have shown that these intensive diabetes treatments are essential in reducing the risk of micro- and macrovascular complications (small and large blood vessel disease which can lead to stroke and heart disease). Therefore, intensive diabetes regimes will prove ineffective if the individual does not wish to (or is unable to) improve their diabetes self-management.

As we have seen, simply having knowledge of the consequences of poor diabetes self-management, and the skills and motivation to assess potential health risks does not necessarily mean that the individual can effectively self-manage their condition. Diabetes education has been criticised for presuming that an increase in information automatically increases knowledge, thus encouraging the individual's self-care and self-management behaviour towards concordance with medical advice (Golin, et al., 2001). The distinction between attitude change and behaviour change means that one does not equal the other. As a result, Hall, et al. (2003) suggested that a change must occur in both the individual's attitude and behaviour in order for them to manage their condition for the right reasons. This appears simplistic, however, when considering factors such as acceptance of the condition, health beliefs, social situation, depression, disability, or a combination of these resulting in poor health outcomes which are inextricably linked and which the individual cannot control.

Locus of control

This is a term applied to a 'personality difference' which influences the individual's perception of a stressful event and its impact on behaviour (Burns, 2001). The individual's locus of control is the degree of control that they have over a situation or event, therefore a person who has a high degree of control over a situation is less likely to become stressed by it. This degree of control is termed an internal locus because the individual has control over their environment and they can direct their existence to a certain degree. A major determinant of stress and emotion is the individual's knowledge of his or her ability to control a situation. Those who do not feel as though they have any control over what happens to them because their lives are dictated by or subject to other people's action conversely have an external locus of control.

Thus, stress is far more influential in the lives of those with an external locus and may actually reach harmful levels if the individual feels that they can do absolutely nothing about a stressful situation. This state of mind was termed 'learned helplessness' by Seligman (1975), who also attributed some forms of depression to this state of mind. This occurs when the individual finds that they are in a situation where their responses are irrelevant to that situation, or where there is no correct response, or where inappropriate responses have been learned (Burns, 2001). Over time, and when this behaviour is applied to different situations, the individual believes that they are unable to cope with the world. Seligman addressed this successfully with positive encouragement for the individual to succeed at small tasks, gradually progressing to more complex ones.

When applied to diabetes, the loss of control over health and blood glucose levels may cause the individual to feel unable to manage the condition successfully, especially if it is brittle Type 1 diabetes. Individuals learn from successful past experience if they believe that the success was based on skill and not luck. It is also the case that the individual will cope better with stress if they believe they have some control over the outcome: their diabetes control and management. Learned helplessness – believing that there is nothing that can be done about a difficult situation, such as having a chronic condition that demands continual self-management – often leads to depression, anxiety and hostility because the individual loses their initiative. It is therefore important for diabetes health professionals to recognise these tendencies and offer support for the individual to achieve small steps in diabetes self-management to boost confidence and escape a situation of learned helplessness.

Motivation and health beliefs
Motivation has been defined in psychological terms as, 'consisting of internal processes that spur us on to satisfy some need' (Burns, 2001; Sheldon, et al., 2000). It has also been explained more simply as the reason for action, or asking, 'what is my motive?', and the reason for that action,

or asking, 'how motivated am I?' (Dixon, 2008). The reason we carry out our actions are multiple and as such, many opinions have been put forward about how motivation operates. Some theories emphasise goal-setting and conscious decision-making, but few theories have tried to combine these concepts of motivation (West, 2006).

Probably the best known theory of motivation in human behaviour is Maslow's (1943) Hierarchy of Needs model, which proposes the acquisition of knowledge and understanding, emphasising the individual's role in achieving their own physical, social and cultural needs as a path to knowledge. Maslow distinguished these needs in order of importance so that physiological needs are a priority before safety needs. The individual's needs in this model are stacked in a pyramid, with a broad base being formed by physiological needs. As the pyramid rises, safety needs come next, followed by love and belonging, self-esteem, self-actualisation, and finally the intellectual needs of understanding and knowledge. For those with diabetes, Maslow's theory implies that health professionals will be unable to impart knowledge to the patient unless the individual's emotional needs are addressed first. Because motivation is necessary to achieve a reachable goal, motivation for diabetes self-care is driven by success, creating a cyclical process, so that motivation enables the behaviour and the success of that behaviour creates the motivation to do it again (self-efficacy). As previously mentioned, empowerment has been cited as the key to this process, through knowledge, control, and the ability to implement decisions.

It has been suggested that motivation can be internal or external, explaining the desire an individual has to undertake an activity without receiving a reward – the motivation coming from satisfaction at feeling competent and self-determined (Deci and Ryan, 2000). Motivation is therefore influenced by both conscious and sub-conscious means; internal and external drives; the individual's beliefs about the consequences of their actions; the perceived outcome of any change in behaviour; and the attitudes and approval of others.

The Health Belief model (Becker and Janz, 1985) was applied specifically to the degree of motivation an individual has for their diabetes self-care, and proposes four different levels of concordance and motivation, ranging from non-concordance to complete diligence and achievement of good self-management behaviour. They concluded that the individual bases their behaviour on their perception of the severity of their diabetes, therefore the amount of self-care activity an individual is prepared to engage in related to their belief that preventative action will reduce the threat of poor control of diabetes. However, as we have already seen, the level of motivation for different self-care activities varies, meaning that some behaviours are conducted more regularly than others, and this changes with the individual's circumstances. This can be seen in a study by Horne (1997) who showed that specific health beliefs and behaviours are related to the ability to manage diabetes treatment demands, suggesting that older individuals, those with secondary chronic complications such as sight difficulties, or those with a long-duration of the condition have impaired motivation for diabetes self-care.

In terms of health beliefs, the perceived susceptibility to diabetes and its chronic complications may be both a motivating and a de-motivating factor, as well as clarifying the perceived benefits of carrying out self-care activities. The following quotes demonstrate this issue:

> I think complications are bound to happen anyway because the body doesn't deal with glucose in the same way if you've got diabetes. Also, I know that some people develop complications even with good glucose control, and others don't even though their sugars are often high.

> No matter how much time and effort I invest in my diabetes management, I can't get good blood glucose control.

Negative health beliefs are clearly a barrier to achieving good diabetes control and management. Although a specific diabetes health belief scale has been reported by some researchers in the past (Bradley, 1994; Jenny, 1984; Given, et al., 1983), problems have been encountered when trying to apply this model to diabetes as a chronic disease. This was the case because the compliance approach dominated how diabetes self-care was measured thirty-plus years ago, rather than the current patient-centred approach, where diabetes care is tailored to the patient's needs.

It is also the case that diabetes self-care is difficult to monitor by outsiders because it relies on self-reporting by the patient, and the individual's beliefs are modified by changes to their behaviour, so the resulting belief is actually a result of the behaviour after the outcome is achieved. Therefore, this may not be the same as the belief that predicted the behaviour and perhaps predicted the change. Ultimately, this may lead to the individual reverting to previous and less-healthy diabetes management behaviour, resulting in poorer glycaemic control. Broome and Llewelyn (1995) have argued that the predictive power of the individual's health beliefs in chronic disease may be naturally limited because of this feedback loop. In addition, in order for patients to achieve a certain level of self-management behaviour, they have to become aware of this by the provision of information and diabetes education.

Although still prior to the favoured patient-centred approach to diabetes care, Glasgow, et al. (1999) used the concept of perceived susceptibility in an attempt to predict those patients who would successfully adopt diabetes self-care behaviours. The researchers found that the patients' health beliefs did not predict all aspects of self-care and self-management activity. Significant correlations were found between active self-care behaviours and self-monitoring of blood glucose, but not for other outcomes, such as exercise and diet. However, the authors did state that there were distinct differences between the perceived benefits of health regime concordance for those with long-duration diabetes, and for older individuals. Whilst this study is not current, it does highlight the difficulty of applying models of behaviour to diabetes regime concordance because of the number of variables, such as age, duration of diabetes, and chronic complications that must be accounted for in the effects.

Self-confidence

Self-confidence is the same as self-efficacy – the concept proposed by the HBM to mean the individual's confidence to carry out a specific positive health behaviour. Dixon (2008) has suggested that an individual's confidence may be significantly reduced because they fear the consequences of trying something new, if they have had previous experience of failure (for example, giving up smoking), or if their emotional/mental state presents barriers (for example, depression and anxiety). Bandura's (1977a, 1997b) concept of self-efficacy fails to recognise these barriers to behaviour change as it suggests that the individual is able to undertake a certain behaviour regardless of the circumstances or context. A similar concept exists in the Theory of Planned Behaviour – a further concept of the Theory of Reasoned Action – describing the extent to which the individual believes they have control over an aspect of their behaviour or a certain action (Azjen, 1985; Dixon, 2008).

Self-confidence and motivation are intrinsically linked to an individual's intention to undertake a specific behaviour, whether it be giving up smoking or doing more blood tests each day and acting on the results to self-manage diabetes more effectively. Self-confidence also enables the individual to achieve their goal. Therefore, once the individual has decided to take action, self-efficacy (self-confidence) helps maintain the effort required to overcome any barriers to sustaining that behaviour (Dixon, 2008). It has been suggested that intention to undertake a behaviour is different to planning, initiating or maintaining that behaviour (Sniehotta, et al., 2005), meaning that self-confidence is important at all stages of behavioural change (Wilson, 2009; West, 2006). For diabetes health professionals, the theories that underlie self-efficacy, motivation and behaviour change are important because they can shape interactions with, and interventions for people with the condition.

ENCOURAGING MOTIVATION AND CONFIDENCE

There are few interventions designed to encourage motivation and confidence in health behaviour, and even fewer aimed specifically at diabetes self-care. Dixon (2008) has suggested that interventions based on particular theoretical models that aim to address issues of motivation and confidence only impact on behaviour and not the components that make up that behaviour, such as self-efficacy or motivation. Bandura (2000), in his Social Cognitive Theory, has suggested that self-efficacy can be enhanced by tackling barriers to behaviour change in manageable stages; observing and learning from the successful change in others that the individual regards as similar to him or herself; and possessing a positive mental attitude that success can be attained, whilst avoiding stress and negative emotions using relaxation exercises.

Interventions based on the Stages of Change model (Prochaska and DiClemente, 1984) have been criticised as varying widely with regard to enabling behaviour change as in practice, some interventions only provided tailored information, whilst others employed goal-setting or relapse-prevention strategies (Dixon, 2008). Because of the varying inclusion of certain concepts under the umbrella of the Stages of Change model, the effectiveness of these strategies has often been poor. Littell and Girvin (2002) questioned the validity of the SoC approach after reviewing 87 studies which reported the application of the SoC to a range of health behaviours, showing minimal change had been achieved.

Rollnick (2000) proposed the technique of motivational interviewing: a patient-centred technique designed to prepare an individual for behavioural change, also called brief negotiation (Rollnick and Miller, 2002). This approach is used more often in the United States than in the UK to coach people who have chronic illness, addictions, or those who wish to modify their health behaviour (Dixon, 2008). Motivational interviewing is a two-phase approach, focussing on building motivation for change and strengthening commitment to change. A plan is then negotiated and the commitment may be shared with others to enable support for change (Miller and Rollnick, 2002). Whilst there have been a number of trials using this method in smoking cessation, few have reported success (Dixon, 2008). Burke, et al. (2002) showed that brief negotiation had a short-lived effect over alternative treatments in two studies targeting diet and exercise behaviour; and two studies which showed brief negotiation had a marked effect in improving control when used in conjunction with an existing medical regime. A systematic review of motivational inter-viewing studies targeting the same behaviour showed that the results varied greatly, and that any effects were minimal (Hettima, et al., 2005).

Self-Regulation Theory and Control Theory are two further inter-ventions where goal-setting and action planning are utilised in order to change behaviour. Locke and Latham (2002) have stated that this approach focusses on personally-defined goals rather than a goal set by a health professional for the individual to aspire to. Self-Regulation Theory suggests that the individual reflects on their progress and feeds this information back to the health professionals providing their care because it can help to maintain a change in weight or blood pressure. However, this reflection of outcomes and focus on the need to achieve an improvement may actually be de-motivating if blood glucose levels are not improved, despite increasing self-care. For example, blood glucose levels tend to be higher if the individual is stressed or depressed due to the biological and psychological factors affecting glucose metabolism. Depression interacts negatively with diabetes (Clark, 2004), leading to erratic diabetes control and a 1.8 percent increase in HbA1c (Mazze, et al., 1984).

Targeting behaviours to achieve change
Interventions must be designed specifically to target a single behaviour and employ measures to overcome that behaviour, such as addiction, in order to be successful. In terms of diabetes care, there are no specific interventions to target poor self-care behaviour as individual health education tends to be employed. For those with Type 2 diabetes which has developed predominantly due to obesity (where insulin cannot act

correctly due to the presence of fat in the body cells), interventions to target obesity may be of value. Slevin (2004) suggested that individuals who received intensive counselling about behavioural intention achieved a greater weight loss than those who did not.

Avenell et al (2006) have suggested that reverse psychology may be employed in encouraging physical activity, where emphasis is placed on decreasing physical inactivity rather than increasing activity. This is achieved by incorporating physical activity into the individual's every day activities (such as taking the stairs rather than the lift) and using prompts and reminders to change behaviour via frequent contact with health professionals. Again, this could be viewed as de-motivating if the individual is not achieving an increase in physical activity and it also relies on self-reporting of behaviour change.

Once an individual becomes aware that they could potentially change their behaviour, possibly via the trigger of a diabetes education message, their intention changes so that they can chose to adopt the new or altered behaviour. Webb and Sheeran (2006) looked at how powerful the intention is in forcing behaviour change by measuring studies providing information about the behaviour and its outcome, risk awareness litera-ture, skill enhancement strategies and goal setting activities. The results showed that a medium to large change in intention only resulted in a small to medium change in behaviour. As would be expected, there was less impact from the intention when the individual had less control over the behaviour, for example, the intention to lose weight and exercise more in Type 1 diabetes when hypoglycaemia is frequent and unexpected. This determines that the individual has to eat or drink more sweet foods to correct blood glucose levels. It is also the case that when hypoglycaemia is severe, the individual over-eats as the brain tries to protect itself from a lack of glucose that it needs for fuel, meaning that the individual is ravenously hungry and consumes a vast amount of carbohydrate-rich calories (Wilson, 2014).

It is clear that the main barrier to change is the individual themselves: once a change in health behaviour is decided upon, the process can begin. Whilst a trigger factor such as a health education message or intervention may be the reason the individual decides to take action, this decision must be the individual's. Behavioural change interventions on their own are unlikely to make any impact on the individual's health outcomes if that person is unwilling to change, or has not reached a stage allowing them to make this decision. Dixon (2008) has stated that there appears to be little clarity about which techniques or interventions work, other than that the individual must be motivated to make a change and be confident that they can achieve that change.

BEHAVIOUR CHANGE IN DIABETES: WHY AND HOW?

As we have seen, health professionals will assess the best way to help the individual implement effective diabetes self-management behaviours by taking into account a multitude of factors. The individual must be aware of what they will gain from engaging in appropriate diabetes self-management behaviour. This depends on their motivation and attitude rather than their knowledge and skills alone. The theoretical framework for diabetes education must then recognise the issues, goals, motivations and perceived barriers that are important to the person with diabetes, and these are unique to that individual. The Stages of Change approach has been applied to many groups of people because it is applicable to all stages of readiness for change. Diabetes interventions which aim to improve glycaemic control have provided guidance on the clinical management of diabetes (the Diabetes Control and Complications Trial, 1993) but there is little guidance relating to how or why people are able to change.

The author conducted telephone interviews with 10 proactive individuals with Type 1 diabetes taking either multiple daily insulin injections (MDI) or using insulin pump therapy treatment – five females and five males of varying ages and durations of diabetes living across the UK – to examine whether their communication with health professionals influenced behaviour change (Wilson, 2009). The individuals were asked a series of questions regarding whether diabetes services had helped them improve their glycaemic control and diabetes self-management; whether they had changed the way they managed their diabetes using intensive methods; what motivated them to change; who helped them make the changes; and whether it was difficult to maintain the change in their lifestyle. The responses were then assessed to identify the stage of change in the SoC model that they most related to: pre-contemplation, contemplation, planning, action, or maintenance.

It was found that contemplation, maintenance or relapse of diabetes self-management behaviours occurred for different reasons according to treatment type. Two of the individuals taking MDI were motivated to improve their glycaemic control in order to progress to insulin pump therapy. However, this is contradictory because pump therapy is often suggested and initiated by a diabetes consultant because MDI fails to keep blood glucose levels stable (NICE, 2003). This means that good control of blood glucose could be achieved with MDI if the individual engaged in the correct behaviour. This involves frequent blood testing (six times per day), acting on the results to see where more or less insulin is needed and taking the correct dose of insulin at the right time to work during meals, and so as not to overlap with a previous insulin dose. The two individuals who relapsed back to their previous diabetes care behaviour provided the following comments:

> When I was getting ready to change to a pump in my mind, I was different about my diabetes. I did more blood tests and watched what I ate and drank... The clinic then thought [I didn't] need the aid of a pump... [That] was about six months ago. I don't feel motivated anymore.

> I found it was very demanding to constantly be testing my blood; watching what I ate; calculating how much insulin I needed; when it was taken etc., and trying to fit that in with everything else

I have to do in my life, like work and the kids. It was virtually impossible – a full-time job!

Individuals taking MDI and those using pump therapy both planned to take on improved diabetes self-management behaviours which were enabled by their primary care health professionals and the flexibility offered by intensive diabetes treatment methods. They gave the following comments:

> I think my doctor feels I know more about my diabetes than I actually do, but he does provide good information. He makes me feel comfortable in discussing changes to my diet and exercise regime, and I always go to him if I need any help with my diabetes, rather than my consultant who is always very busy.

> I had been wanting to get better blood sugar results for a while, and when I had my annual diabetes clinic appointment I discussed it with my diabetes nurse, who helped me with good suggestions and support.

All of the pump users had already adapted to a treatment change, on average for 5–13 years before this study was conducted, so their improved diabetes management behaviour was firmly embedded into their routine. Some of those taking MDI found it easier than others to take more exercise and alter their injection timings to incorporate this change into their lifestyle:

> My Practice Nurse told me that I needed to have a little bit of insulin even if I was exercising because the liver releases glucose to the muscles which can put blood sugar levels up. I also now test my blood glucose before exercising to make sure I'm not too low, or too high, as that can put a strain on the heart. I now feel able to tackle exercise more regularly and enjoy it without worry.

> I tend to eat a lot more when I'm depressed and take more insulin to cover the increase in blood glucose. I wanted to stop doing this, but found I couldn't. My nurse suggested I do more blood tests to

see how high I was going and to try and count the carbohydrates of the foods so I had enough insulin to cover it, so that helps.

All of the five pump users had also been able to maintain their use of this intensive insulin treatment due to the knowledge that by keeping blood glucose levels stable, they were being proactive in preventing or delaying the worsening of existing chronic complications of diabetes:

> I have mild retinopathy and, since using pump therapy to treat my diabetes, the eye condition has stayed stable for seven years now. This motivates me to continue to use it and do frequent blood glucose tests.

The five pump users also appeared to possess a high level of perceived self-efficacy in managing their diabetes and maintaining this behaviour, as the following comment demonstrates:

> I have mastered the use of pump therapy because it is a technology that helps me have control over my Type 1 diabetes, rather than it having control over me.

Intensive self-management of diabetes requires the individual to be proactive and highly motivated to maintain the adoption of MDI or pump therapy in order to prevent, reduce, or stabilise chronic complications. The cited small study demonstrates that this was the case for the five pump users taking part. These highly motivated individuals also needed the advice and support of health professionals to enable them to progress to and maintain a state of effective diabetes self-management. This was highlighted by the person who relapsed and lost motivation for self-care after his efforts led to an insulin pump being denied because it was decided he could achieve the same effect on blood glucose with multiple insulin injections. These examples show that the individual must be ready for change and that they must want to change their behaviour.

The five MDI users each contemplated and planned to make a change to their self-management behaviour, but were perhaps less able to progress to the action stage to achieve an improvement in glycaemic control because they were using injections, when compared with the flexibility in dosage adjustment that can be achieved with pump therapy (Wilson, 2003b). Each person had reached the contemplation and planning stage of behaviour change, but as well as the person denied a pump after demonstrating improved diabetes control, a second person also experienced a relapse after reaching the action stage. This was due to the perceived demands of acting on frequent blood tests and maintaining the motivation to inject insulin four to six times a day at the correct times and in the correct dosages in order to achieve good control of blood glucose levels. The experiences of these individuals taking MDI demonstrates the cyclical nature of the behaviour change process. Each person had reached their particular stage due to their own motivation, but also the assistance of the health professionals involved in their diabetes care. The health professionals and the varying stages of behaviour change achieved were:

- Diabetes team including a clinical psychologist – action then relapse
- General Practitioner – contemplation then planning
- Practice Nurse – contemplation and planning/action
- Diabetes consultant – maintenance
- Diabetes team – action then relapse

The five people using insulin pump therapy had maintained their use of the technology because of perceived vulnerability to complications and a high degree of self-efficacy. Initial information from their GP, diabetes team, or family and friends with diabetes triggered their motivation to contact the insulin pump manufacturer or the Insulin Pump Therapy (INPUT) national voluntary diabetes organisation for information. For those who did not hear about pump therapy treatment via a health professional, this was possibly because the individual was not felt to have a clinical need for the treatment to be initiated (the criteria being frequent and unpredictable hypoglycaemia and or an inability to manage diabetes with MDI in order to prevent/stabilise chronic complications). None of the pump users stated that they had relapsed back to MDI due to poor glycaemic control or an inability to incorporate the intensive demands of pump therapy into their lifestyle.

This study involved individuals who were already motivated to change their diabetes self-management behaviour demonstrating, as previously suggested, that the individual must want to change and be ready for change. This indicates that the wider population of people with diabetes often do not engage in appropriate self-care behaviours because they are not at a state of readiness for change, or because they have not been triggered into making changes. Some of the individuals in this small study were more motivated than others, enabling those proactive people to maintain their use of insulin pump therapy treatment because of the benefits of flexibility and control of glucose levels. Adopting intensive self-management behaviour to achieve and maintain normal glycaemic control to prevent complications has not been shown to be the case for the wider diabetes population (Ruggiero, 2000). The findings from the author's small study indicate the importance of a positive alteration in the individual's behaviour as well as in their attitude towards their diabetes self-management. Insulin pump therapy users were able to change their behaviour because it is enabled by the available technology and specific information, education and support provided by a number of sources (Wilson 2009; 2003b).

CHAPTER 2

DIABETES AND DEPRESSION

In 1992, The Global Burden of Disease Study was jointly instigated by the World Health Organisation, the World Bank, and Harvard University to evaluate the burden of 100 common diseases. This study clearly demonstrated the global impact of neuropsychiatric illness (Murray and Lopez, 1997). Depression was shown to be the fourth leading cause of disability in the world and was predicted to become the second leading cause of disability by 2020. In developed countries, major depression was already a primary cause of disease burden, exceeding all other diseases except ischemic heart disease (due to blocked arteries and poor blood supply). To put this into context, Murray and Lopez (1996) have equated the degree of disability conferred by depression as equal to the functional impairment from blindness or paraplegia.

Studies show that over 90 percent of individuals who commit suicide had suffered from depression, substance abuse, or another serious mental disorder (Williams, et al., 2006; Preskorn, 1999). There are also studies that have found a correlation between the burden and severity of comorbid medical illness (two or more conditions being present at the same time), such as depression and diabetes, and suicide (Ikeda, et al., 2001). Depression is also associated with increased medical morbidity (how often a disease occurs) and mortality (the number of deaths from a given cause). For example, Carney and Freedland (2003) found that patients with depression who had suffered a myocardial infarction (destruction of a portion of the myocardium of the heart due to poor or absent blood supply) had a significantly elevated risk of future coronary events and death compared to non-depressed patients.

A further analysis of 25 studies by Cuijpers and Smit (2002) found that depression increases mortality from all causes, with the relative risk of dying being 1.8 times higher in depressed individuals compared to non-depressed persons. These studies highlight the extensive adverse effects of untreated depression, whether undiagnosed or due to patient non-concordance, with an emphasis on the individual's decreased capacity and functioning, and the heightened risk of suicide and death from all causes.

EFFECTS OF DEPRESSION

Undoubtedly the presence of depression adversely affects diabetes both physiologically and psychologically. It negatively influences the individual reporting any symptoms associated with their diabetes. It also reduces the individual's concordance with health professional's advice and their diabetes self-care behaviour which leads to prolonged poor glycaemic control. This in turn significantly increases the risk of developing chronic long-term complications of diabetes, such as blindness, limb amputation and kidney failure (De Groot, et al., 2001; UK Prospective Diabetes Study Group, 1998; Karlson and Agardh, 1997; Diabetes Control and Complications Trial, 1993). The effects of depression in an individual with diabetes are many and should not be under-estimated by either the individual or by health professionals.

The reason why people with diabetes also frequently suffer from depression is unconfirmed but Clark (2004) has suggested that it results from psychological, physical and genetic factors. Evidence is conflicting with regard to whether depression is an independent risk factor for diabetes (Brown, et al., 2005; Carthenon, et al., 2003; Saydah, et al., 2003). A number of psychological and physical changes occur in people with diabetes, including neurochemical and neurovascular abnormalities and there is evidence to suggest that genetic factors may have a role despite the fact that they are unrelated to diabetes (Chiba, et al., 2000; Lustman, et al., 1997a; 1992). The contribution of these factors is different for each individual but the necessity of adopting lifestyle changes, adjustments for dietary restriction and treatment regime, and coping with the ongoing necessity of diabetes self-care, for example, regular self-monitoring of blood glucose, takes its toll. Physical impairment due to chronic complications of diabetes such as sight loss (diabetic retinopathy) or dealing with chronic nerve pain due to diabetic neuropathy also impacts heavily on mental health status.

Among patients with diabetes in primary care, 4–15 percent meet the criteria for major depression and another 9–16 percent meet the criteria for a diagnosis of other psychological disorders such as anxiety (Tiemens, et al., 1996; Williams, et al., 1995). Elderly and poor individuals have particularly high rates of depression, and these groups also are at greatest risk for diabetes and diabetes-related complications (Piette, et al., 2004; De Groot, et al., 2001; Singh, et al., 2001). Depression is three times more prevalent in individuals with diabetes when compared with the general population, affecting at least 15 percent of the diabetes population (Clark, 2004; Gavard, et al., 1993; Peyrot, et al, 1997). It is also more prevalent in patients with diabetes and other chronic health conditions such as arthritis (Pouwer, et al., 2003). Just over one-third (33 percent) of people with diabetes have an episode of major depression in their lifetime, a figure higher than for the general population (Clark, 2004; Lustman, et al., 1998a). It is also the case that after an initial episode of depression, patients with diabetes relapse more frequently than other patients (Clark, 2004; Lustman, et al., 1997b).

THE PHYSICAL AND HEALTHCARE COSTS OF DEPRESSION

Severe depression has a major impact on all aspects of the individual's health and social situation. This includes functional disability and absenteeism from work, college or school, as well as increased healthcare expenditure (Clark, 2004). Lustman, et al. (1998b) have suggested that depression in persons with diabetes is recurrent and more severe than in the general population and that less than 10 percent of individuals with remission from diabetes-related depression remain symptom free for longer than 5 years. Further studies have shown that depression occurs more often in women with diabetes than in men with the condition which is equally true in the general population, and that rates of depression are similar in those with Type 1 and Type 2 diabetes (Anderson, et al., 2001; Talbot and Nouwen, 2000; Gavard, et al., 1993). Anderson, et al. (2001) have estimated that having diabetes therefore doubles the chance of also developing depression.

Because of the debilitating nature of depression, it reacts adversely with diabetes. It is the case that the brain relies on glucose as its primary source of fuel, but if there is hyper- or hypoglycaemia, normal brain function is impeded. A number of studies have linked high blood glucose levels and depression, where as little as a 1.8 percent increase in HbA1c (glycosylated haemoglobin – the amount of glucose sticking to the red blood cells over a three-month period) has been shown to cause depressive symptoms (Mazze, et al., 1984); and the UK Prospective Diabetes Study (1998a; 1998b) found that 49 percent of insulin-treated patients and 56 percent of those treated with diabetes medication had HbA1c values of 8.0 percent or higher (6.0 to 6.5 percent being the recommendation in the UK and an average of <7.0 percent in the United States). Depression is therefore both a condition in its own right and a complication of diabetes and it is exacerbated by poor glycaemic control in the same way that physical complications such as eye disease (retinopathy), nerve damage (neuropathy), kidney impairment (nephropathy) and circulatory system complications are triggered or worsened.

It is also the case that depression has been directly linked to the development of neuropathy and cardiovascular disease (Clark, 2004), having direct and indirect links to glycaemic control and diabetes complications in adults (De Groot, et al., 2001; Lustman, et al., 1992) and adolescents (La Greca, et al., 1995). The link between depression, glycaemic control and complications can be seen in the following comment from a sufferer:

> I've noticed that when I'm depressed my neuropathy in my feet and legs is worse, even if my blood glucose levels seem OK. It is especially bad at night, with sharp pains in my calves and periodic prickling and numbness in the soles of my feet. It isn't continuous pain, but it will keep happening five or six times in the night with sharp little jabs; enough to keep me awake, which makes me feel even worse.

Having depression is also a risk factor for developing high blood pressure – hypertension (Davidson, et al., 2000), increased levels of harmful blood fats – hyperlipidaemia (Gary, et al., 2000), and heart failure (Abramson, et al, 2001), and each of these conditions increases the rate of cardiovascular events among patients with diabetes. The reason why these conditions contribute towards heart disease may differ for patients with type 1 and type 2 diabetes (Ciechanowski, et al., 2003) although as we have already seen, depression is associated with poor glycaemic control (Lutman, et al., 2000) which is undoubtedly the underlying factor.

Symptoms such as tiredness, increased thirst, frequent urination, blurred vision, slow healing of wounds, numbness in the feet and legs, and obesity may be tolerated by the individual for many years before consulting a doctor. It is known that Type 2 diabetes may remain undiagnosed for up to 12 years (Diabetes UK, 2008), meaning that hyperglycaemia is prolonged and untreated, perhaps explaining the prevalence of heart disease in this group. Patients with diabetes and depression also have higher rates of retinopathy (De Groot, et al., 2001; Cohen, et al., 1997) and macrovascular complications such as stroke than diabetes patients without depression (De Groot, et al., 2001; Hannien, et al.,

1999); and depressed patients report more diabetes-related symptoms (Ciechanowski, et al., 2003).

Inactivity and obesity are also associated with depression, as well as non-concordance with the diabetes treatment regime and the advice of health professionals. These lifestyle factors and consequences also impact negatively on glycaemic control. For this reason,

interventions such as smoking cessation programmes centred on changing the individual's lifestyle, are not successful as lifestyle change requires motivation and self-efficacy fuelled by a desire to want to improve health status. Anderson, et al. (2001) has suggested that depression may oppose efforts to achieve good glycaemic control and that the condition is clinically relevant in almost one out of every three patients with diabetes. This could be due to the effect depression has on metabolic control in diabetes, making it very difficult to achieve blood glucose levels within the normal range.

The view that behavioural interventions are ineffective in terms of addressing depression is supported by DiMatteo, et al., 2000; Littlefield, et al., 1992, and McGill, et al., 1992; and that physiological interventions are equally unsatisfactory (Jacobson and Sapolsky, 1991; Young, et al., 1991; Levy, et al., 1983; Ettigi, et al., 1977). Successful treatment of depression is therefore strongly associated with improvements in glycaemic control (Lustman, et al., 1998b; De Rubeis, et al., 1990). Because of the difficulties of matching a suitable treatment approach to the patient's needs, medical conditions and current prescribed medications, the condition often goes undiagnosed, and two of every three cases of depression are left untreated by primary care physicians (Lustman and Harper, 1987). The following comment demonstrates a patient's experience of living with depression and diabetes:

> I have had depression for nearly 40 years since I was diagnosed with Type 1 diabetes. I have been prescribed medication that made me feel like a zombie; I've seen several psychiatrists – one who said he could see no reason why I was depressed as I

was dressed cheerfully; and I've undergone several months of Cognitive Behavioural Therapy to address my thought patterns and behaviours, and to encourage me to set goals – all of these didn't work. I was told by one clinical psychologist that if I wanted to kill myself, then I should do so because it was my choice and it would make me really think about it. So now, when I get sucked back down into depression again, I just don't mention it to my GP or anyone really because no one can do anything to help and most don't even understand.

Hanninen, et al. (1999) and Jacobson, et al. (1997) have suggested that depression directly affects the quality of life of patients coping with chronic illness, including diabetes. Depression is known to cause adverse effects in individuals with cardiac disorders and stroke, increasing the mortality rate among these patients (Vaccarino, et al., 2001; Jonas and Mussolino, 2000; Frasure-Smith, et al., 1993). Because of its effect on the mental rather than physical health of the individual, depression compromises every aspect of life more than physical health conditions such as high blood pressure, chronic lung diseases, gastrointestinal disorders and arthritis (Druss, et al., 2000; Schulberg, et al., 1988). Although studies by Lustman (2000b; 1998b) have shown that glycaemic control is only slightly improved by the treatment of depression and in one case was significantly worsened (Lustman, 1997), the patient's quality of life is undoubtedly improved by the remission of depressive symptoms.

A correlation has been found between depression in patients with diabetes and an increase in reported functional limitations (Ciechanowski, et al., 2003; 2000). For this reason, an increase in physical activity may be an effective form of behavioural change for patients with diabetes and depression as other research has shown a link between physical inactivity, depression and diabetes (Piette, et al., 2004; Biddle, et al., 2000; Hassmen, et al., 2000). It is to be expected that individuals with diabetes who are physically active have better metabolic control and therefore experience fewer depressive symptoms or even have a faster recovery from an episode of major depression. Further studies have confirmed this, reiterating the knowledge that reduced physical activity majorly increases the risk of depression (Biddle, et al., 2000; Camacho, et al., 1991; Farmer, et al., 1988).

Whilst depression has a severe impact on motivation, and interventions to treat the depression itself have been suggested as ineffective, it has been shown that exercise programmes for people with diabetes and depression are beneficial. Boule, et al. (2001) found that individuals participating in these exercise programmes had an average HbA1c level of 7.7 percent compared with 8.3 percent for the comparison group who did not exercise. The benefits of taking regular moderate exercise was also shown to reduce cardiovascular risk factors such as high-density lipoprotein (HDL blood fat levels), cholesterol and blood pressure levels. Similar findings were shown for patients with major depression who undertook a four-month course of either aerobic exercise, anti-depressant medication, or a combination of exercise and anti-depressant therapy (Blumenthal, et al., 1999). After 10 months, those in the exercise group were assessed to be 30 percent less likely to have had a depressive relapse than those in the medication group (Babyak, et al., 2000). In addition, Singh, et al. (2001) conducted a study looking at depression in elderly individuals. The researchers found that regular exercise resulted in the participants being 50 percent less likely to have depression after 5 months of increased physical activity than participants in a similar group who did not exercise. These studies show that exercise is a crucial component in treating and managing depression, especially where the suspected cause is hyperglycaemia in patients with diabetes.

As previously mentioned, depression in diabetes leads to poor glycaemic control because of a combination of metabolic changes and, frequently, the individual's disinterest in diabetes self-care activities. This manifests as behavioural characteristics such as negative thought processes, internalising (having an internal rather than an external locus of control) and pessimistic attributional styles (consistently blaming oneself for negative things that happen), and displaying passive (emotionally-focussed) rather than proactive coping strategies (Goodman and Whitaker, 2002; Abramson, et al., 2001; Beck, et al., 1979). Negative thought patterns also cause depressed patients to expect negative events to repeat themselves with the same adverse results. Individuals with diabetes who have experienced negative events may carry this feeling of learned helplessness over into their diabetes self-care, feeling that they are unable to manage their condition effectively due to their depression and situations beyond their control. This mind-set also means that the individual is highly unlikely to follow through any plans for health-related behaviour change as they believe it is unachievable or will be of little value.

Ciechanowski, et al. (2003) and DiMatteo, et al. (2000) have found a causal link between depression and the decreased ability of patients with chronic illness to stick to their self-care routine. Ziegelstein, et al. (2000) studied patients undergoing cardiac rehabilitation and found that individuals with depression were less likely to follow treatment recommendations after a heart attack, including taking prescribed medication. Similarly, Ciechanowski, et al. (2000) found that a group of individuals with Type 2 diabetes who also had depression did not take their blood glucose lowering medication as prescribed half as often as patients with milder or no depressive symptoms. In a further study, patients with diabetes and depressive symptoms experienced more diabetes-related physical symptoms one year later due to their previous poor self-care behaviour (McKellar, et al., 2004). It is known that the complications of diabetes can occur up to ten years after a prolonged period of poor glycaemic control (Shaw and Cummings, 2005). Conversely, patients who have experienced remission of their depression are known to experience a sense of self-efficacy (De Rubeis, et al., 1990) enabling them to increase their diabetes self-care which is associated with improved glycaemic control.

Depression is known to lessen the patient's ability to be able to communicate effectively with health professionals. This type of two-way communication is essential for patients with diabetes and ultimately has an impact on diabetes self-management and glycaemic control as shown in the following comment:

> When I have depression it's like I have a mental block that stops me thinking, remembering what I want to say, being able to discuss something, or even just answering questions my diabetes consultant asks me. I then get angry with myself, especially if I've forced myself to go to the appointment in the first place. There have been a couple of times when I haven't even been able to go along because I think, 'What's the point? He's just going to say I haven't looked after my diabetes very well.' Then this makes me annoyed with my consultant for not recognising my difficulties and helping me, although I was recently told by the diabetes nurse that I need to say what the problem is because my consultant isn't a mind reader.

Satisfaction with the health professional/patient communication process is a strong predictor of concordance with the diabetes medical regime and good metabolic control. Wilson (2003a) found that patient satisfaction with their diabetes care involved many factors, from good communication by and with health professionals to the ability to speak to a consultant or nurse when necessary, and the availability of a counsellor or clinical psychologist as part of the diabetes team to address psychosocial issues.

Patients who perceive that their treatment agenda is often overlooked are less satisfied with their diabetes care. This has also been shown generally, where patients who are not satisfied with their medical care are less likely to follow a treatment regime or medical advice and have poorer outcomes (Marple, et al., 1997). A further study of individuals with diabetes has shown that patients require both good general communication and diabetes-specific communication from the healthcare staff they visit (Piette, et al., 2003). This was also found to be the case by Wilson (2003a) in a study of perceived needs of people with Type 1 diabetes.

There are a number of health professionals a patient with diabetes may be required to see, for example, the ophthalmologist for eye checks and the chiropodist/podiatrist for foot care, as well as the diabetes care team, GP and GP Practice nurse. For those individuals with additional medical conditions, this means more opportunity for communication breakdown as the same information is repeated by the patient to each health professional; often perceived by patients as tiresome and by health professionals as disinterest (Wilson, 2003a). This could also be due to patients with diabetes having high expectations of the knowledge of non-diabetes clinicians who demonstrate that they do not to understand the patient's situation from a diabetes perspective.

Depression may lead to further dissatisfaction with encounters between diabetes patients and health professionals because of negative thought processes or because of poorer communication (Katon, 2003). Kroenke, et al. (1997) have suggested that patients with depression are more likely to have unmet expectations after they have been part of a communication process with health professionals and Haviland, et al. (2001) have stated that depressed patients are also less satisfied with the overall medical care they receive. The following comment demonstrates both these points:

> I go to my appointments because I think they will help me. They don't understand how depression affects me and they haven't got the right attitude or the right thing to say. Usually I end up feeling very upset afterwards because someone has said something insensitive or uncaring like, 'You could do a lot to help yourself by looking after your diabetes'. I've never been offered any practical advice or coping strategies, I'm just left to struggle on my own to try and manage. This makes me very angry as they just don't get it.

From the health professional's perspective, patients with depression who present as the person quoted may be beyond their remit if they are not trained in psychological approaches as their needs are complex. Jackson and Kroenke (1999) have found that primary care providers are more likely to consider patients with depressive or anxiety disorders to be 'difficult,' and that they consequently consider patients who have diabetes and depression or anxiety as 'less able to cope with their diabetes'. Petty, et al. (1991) examined the communication process between diabetes consultants and their patients and concluded that they perceived the patient's depression and/or anxiety was a limiting factor in being able to effectively self-manage their condition. This perception ultimately influenced their communication with patients and also their management style. Such attitudes towards certain patients may be evidence-based according to HbA1c levels and observed poor self-care. It has also been shown that there is a correlation between diabetes patients with a 'dismissive' interpersonal communication style with health professionals and poor metabolic control (Ciechanowski, et al., 2001). The following comment demonstrates this:

> I hate being quizzed about my diabetes and how I look after myself. It's not really something I think about day to day: I just do my injections then forget about it. I saw my consultant not long ago and he asked me a question. I just replied, 'I try not to let my diabetes control my life.' I then got a look of disapproval and was told that my HbA1c was 13 percent.

It has been calculated that depressed patients use more healthcare resources and therefore cost more than non-depressed patients. This is perhaps an obvious conclusion when considering that individuals without healthcare needs may rarely visit their GP, let alone a hospital consultant. Druss, et al. (1999) have stated that the need for care and higher healthcare costs for depressed patients with diabetes may be due to their problems with self-care, poor concordance with treatment advice, and difficult interactions with health professionals. In the United States, Ciechanowski, et al. (2000) found that patients with diabetes and depression had healthcare costs that were 86 percent higher than those of non-depressed patients with diabetes. A further study by Egede, et al. (2002) found that total healthcare costs for patients with diabetes and depression were 4.5 times higher than those for non-depressed diabetes patients, and that the groups differed in treatment costs even after adjusting for patients' demographic characteristics, health insurance, and coexisting illnesses.

IDENTIFYING DEPRESSION IN PEOPLE WITH DIABETES

The diagnosis of major depressive disorder is made when the symptoms occur together, when they are severe, and when they persist daily for a minimum of two weeks (American Psychiatric Association, 2013). Although individual symptoms may vary, generalised sadness for no specific reason and lack of interest in pleasurable activities are key diagnostic signs. The symptoms must be categorised as distressing to the individual, or must cause a decline in social, occupational or other key functions to constitute a diagnosis of depression; symptoms that result from taking illicit drugs or prescription medication, or that arise from bereavement are not counted (Clark, 2004). Unfortunately, the symptoms judged as being due to a medical condition, such as the burden of self-care for diabetes, are also not recognised in making a diagnosis of depression, meaning that the mental and physical toll diabetes takes on the individual is discounted.

Although omitting the symptoms of a medical condition as an indicator of depression appears counter-productive in diagnosing mental health issues in diabetes, it is in place because the symptoms of poorly-controlled diabetes are very similar to those of depression. Feeling constantly 'down', unhappy, listless, tired, poorly motivated, disconnected, withdrawn, and irritable, to name but a few symptoms of both conditions are often ignored by health professionals when patients report them if that individual also has a high HbA1c. Diabetes does not directly cause the key symptoms of depression and this practise avoids the over-diagnosis of depression in the diabetes population, reducing the likelihood of a false-positive diagnosis (Clark, 2004). However, Clark continued that poorly controlled diabetes should not impair the clinician's ability to diagnose depression. Despite this statement, depression in diabetes is recognised and treated in less than a third of patients (Lustman, et al, 2000a).

In spite of the potential worth of treatment, patients with diabetes and depression often experience significant gaps in their depression care (Piette, et al., 2004). As we have already seen regarding patients with diabetes, research has shown that health professionals often fail to detect depression among their patients (Tiemens, et al., 1998; Tiemens, et al., 1996; Simon and Von Korff, 1995) and when the condition is identified, depression-specific treatments often are not initiated (Simon and Von Korff, 1995). Health professionals working in primary care who are treating patients with diabetes may lack expertise in mental health issues or may have insufficient time to fully explore depressive symptoms. It is also the case that Cognitive Behavioural Therapy (CBT) is unavailable in certain areas of the country because of the lack of adequately trained therapists or because it is not prescribed due to perceived limitations on mental health benefits for the patient (Corrigan and McCracken, 1995a; 1995b).

Barriers to recovery
Long-term concordance with medical advice for patients taking medication to treat depression is often poor. Lin, et al. (1995) have reported that in a large managed care organization, 28 percent of patients discontinued their anti-depressant medication within the first month of treatment and that 44 percent discontinued their treatment by the third month. Insurance claim data also suggests that up to 70 percent of patients with medical insurance in the United States failed to collect their 30-day prescriptions in the 6 months following initiation of anti-depressant treatment (Hylan, et al., 1999; Melfi, et al., 1996). Eaton, et al. (1996) have suggested that patients with diabetes and depression feel a certain stigma about 'being observed' in a mental health setting making them less likely to engage in discussion about treatment for their conditions.

Sirey, et al. (2001a) have stated that psychological barriers to treatment, such as perceived stigma and the patient's minimisation of the need for care, can be important obstacles to concordance with taking medication for major depression. Individuals who have mental illness have reported being shunned and avoided by work colleagues and friends (Wahl, 1999). The following comment demonstrates this issue:

> I developed depression and had a lot of problems coping with it.
> My GP suggested I should tell people what I was going through
> as they would understand and make allowances. He was wrong. I
> told a friend I had known for many years and she had even worked
> for a mental health charity at one time, so I thought she would be
> a good person to tell. When I told her it was as though we were
> suddenly strangers. She dropped me like a hot potato and refused
> to have any more contact with me. It was like she thought I was
> disgusting and weak for having depression, as though I'd told her
> I'd murdered someone or something terrible rather than it being
> a medical condition I had no control over.

Hanninen, et al. (1999) have suggested that patients may also be unwilling
to undertake a course of treatment for depression because of concerns
about stigma or any side effects, as shown in the following comment:

> My depression has really affected me and some days, I struggle to
> get out of bed and do the simplest chores. I know this sounds silly,
> but I was referred for CBT by my doctor because she thought it
> would help me manage my diabetes, but I felt ashamed to actually
> go along. I felt like everyone at the doctor's surgery knew why
> I was going to the hospital and I didn't want to share that with
> anyone I knew in case they judged me. If I said I was going to the
> diabetes clinic, it wouldn't have been a problem, but because it
> was a mental health thing it made a big difference as my family,
> friends and colleagues at work don't understand it as they've
> never had depression.

Treatment to bring depression under control is effective in the short-
term. However, treatment may be stopped at this point, either because the
patient's doctor or the individual believes they no longer have depression.
It may also be the case that the patient does not wish to undertake the
treatment, either because they perceive the regime to be complex, due
to medication side-effects, or for other reasons such as stigma and how
others perceive them. Unfortunately, research has shown that as few as
40 percent of patients who have diabetes remain free of major depressive

disorder in the year after successful initial treatment, with recurrence of symptoms frequently accompanied by a deterioration in glycaemic control (Williams, et al., 2006).

Psychological and social circumstances are personal to the individual and may change for the worse as well as the better in accordance with health status as is the case for many other factors, such as relationship breakdown or bereavement. Research by Weiden, et al. (1997) looked at some of these aspects in the context of having a mental health condition and following treatment guidelines. The study found that perceived stigma from others and denial by the patient of their illness were associated majorly with non-concordance in a group of individuals with schizophrenia. It has also been found that older adults who are diagnosed with depression felt highly stigmatised by their illness (Sirey, et al., 2001b), perceiving that they should be able to cope and 'pull themselves together,' making them more likely to discontinue their treatment as they deny the diagnosis.

It would be expected that individuals who have a lower perception of stigma and a higher self-rated severity of illness would be more concordant than those who felt highly stigmatised and who reported a lower severity of illness. Sirey, et al. (2001b) found that emphasising the need for anti-depressant treatment with older individuals enhanced concordance with the treatment regime significantly. Patients who were over 60 years of age were found to be more concordant than younger patients and those with personality disorders, such as schizophrenia, were less likely to follow medical advice about their treatment. Severity of depression, limitations on functioning, or the number of visits to health professionals also did not predict concordance. The expectation of treatment side effects or any distress caused by side effects was not found to predict concordance with medical advice. Similar findings have been seen in studies examining concordance with a diabetes regime, where older individuals and those patients who have developed chronic complications were more concordant than the newly-diagnosed (Donnovan, et al., 2002).

Self-reporting of concordance with both a diabetes regime and with taking anti-depressant medication is often shown to be good when based on pill counts (Myers and Branthwaite, 1992; Ley, 1988). However, self-reports may be unreliable as deception, misunderstanding of the regimen, and poor recall must be accounted for. As previously discussed, the patient's health beliefs about concordance with following a medical regime and in this instance, taking anti-depressant medication correctly, is an important factor in predicting health-related behaviours. The Health Belief Model has been used to describe health behaviours such as the use of preventive health measures and concordance with a medical regime once ill-health is diagnosed in order to restore health or prevent further illness. As we have already seen, the HBM suggests that the patient's perception of the severity of an illness is a major influence on subsequent health behaviour (Janz and Becker, 1984). However, as with the diagnosis of diabetes, the patient may be in denial when they are told they have depression, and this denial may ultimately override the severity of the illness.

A further potential barrier to effective depression management among individuals with diabetes is the lack of a unifying view of the patients' clinical problems that encompasses both diabetes and depression. This may involve a lack of collaboration between diabetes care and mental health services. It may also be the case that the diabetes team is located in the hospital setting whilst mental health services are based in the community, meaning that the two are not working in the same setting. This situation heralds communication difficulties for factors such as having separate patient records and the patient having to repeat information to two different teams of health professionals (Fisher and Ransom, 1997; Katon, et al., 1995). Piette, et al. (2004) have stated that primary care providers often do not appreciate the importance of aggressive depression management for patients' overall health, and that patients often do not draw connections between their depressive symptoms and their ability to manage their diabetes. Although the presentation of depression in those with diabetes is well-documented, as well as the availability of suitable treatments, there is little consensus regarding how these co-existing conditions should be effectively managed.

In addition to the desire not to over-diagnose depression in diabetes that leads to the condition frequently not being recognised, it is important to distinguish depression as a condition in its own right, and not as merely as a complication of diabetes, although both are true. Because depression interacts very negatively with diabetes there is a tendency to treat only the medical rather that the medical and mental health condition. The Beck Depression Inventory (BDI) has been used as a preliminary method in the outpatient setting to identify patients with depressive symptoms (Beck and Beamesderfer, 1974). This 21-question patient-completed survey takes 5–10 minutes to answer by summing ratings for each of the questions. A score of >16 identifies a major depressive disorder and this inventory has determined depression in over 70 percent of patients (Lustman, et al., 1992). It has also been suggested that two particular areas of questioning, for example, 'How have you been feeling recently? Have you been low in spirits?', and, 'Have you been able to enjoy the things you usually enjoy?' can determine up to 95 percent of individuals with major depression (Peveler, et al., 2002). As well as the Beck Depression Inventory, the Center for Epidemiologic Studies Depression Scale is also used to identify depression in patients (Radloff, 1977).

When using both the Beck Depression Inventory and the Center for Epidemiologic Studies in Depression Scale in different research studies, depression prevalence was found to be equal to the number of subjects with scores above a specified value. However, the score used to identify depression in the participants varied across studies, for example, a BDI score of 10 in some studies (Songar, et al., 1993; Leedom, et al., 1991) increased to 13 in a study by Stone, et al., 1984; and 16 in a study by Palinkas, et al., 1991. This is deemed acceptable however as the scores used to identify depression are dependent on the perception of the individual completing the questionnaire, and the clinical setting which the patient is attending (Lustman, et al., 1991; Mulrow, et al., 1995).

TREATMENT AND MANAGEMENT

In the short-term, the individual presenting with both diabetes and major depressive disorder requires specific therapeutic intervention as little improvement is seen with non-specific measures (Williams, et al., 2006). Both psychotherapy and anti-depressant medication are effective for treating depression in people with diabetes (Clark, 2004; Lustman, et al., 2000a; 1998b; 1997c). Medication has an advantage over psychotherapy in primary care because it does not require the time and expertise of a psychotherapist to administer and is lower in cost for the healthcare provider. However, in contrast, some anti-depressant medications have undesirable side-effects which are known to exacerbate the difficulties of managing diabetes effectively.

Diabetes management guidelines only provide a framework for treatment of the primary condition (diabetes) and not coexisting conditions such as depression. Depression comes under the broad area of tailoring the guidelines to the individual's specific needs. Unfortunately, this often fails to integrate all care needs, prioritising treatment interventions to target conditions such as depression, and delivery of treatment that incorporates multiple conditions in a way that maximises the patient's wellbeing. This is the medical model of care, where the patient's diabetes is treated as a part of the individual rather than how the diabetes affects the whole patient. This method of delivering diabetes care is now supposedly outmoded as patient-centred care is the norm. However, the identification and treatment of depression and its impact on diabetes self-care often relies on self-reporting, meaning that the full extent of the problem goes unrecognised by health professionals, especially when different health-care teams are involved. This issue is shown by the following comments:

> I have repeatedly told my GP and diabetes consultant that I am suffering from depression and that's why my blood glucose levels are not good. I know that it's depression because I've suffered from it on and off all my life and I know how debilitating it is. Obviously sometimes I have months that are worse than others,

but I get the impression that I'm not being listened to and that the GP and diabetes team don't talk to one another. They think I'm just using my depression as an excuse not to look after my diabetes properly. I always get a lecture on why reducing my glucose levels is important from my GP and my diabetes consultant. I know why my diabetes isn't well-controlled, I just can't do it.

When I moved to a different area I explained to my new diabetes consultant that I have depression. He then looked at me as though I was lying, flicked through my clinic notes and told me I should try harder to look after my diabetes. He had no help to offer and suggested I go to my new GP for some better [anti-depressive] treatment. The GP hadn't even told him I'd got depression. It feels like the consultant doesn't recognise my problem and how it affects my diabetes. Surely I can't be the first person he's ever seen that has diabetes and depression at the same time?

It is clear that depression affects the individual with diabetes by severely impairing their health-related quality of life, reducing physical activity levels, limiting concordance with diabetes self-care regimes, and by impairing the individual's ability to communicate effectively with health professionals (Piette, et al., 2004). A treatment plan for depression should ideally be best-suited to the individual's needs after a full assessment and should involve the patient's partner and key family members. However, this is dependent on resources and availability may vary widely from area to area. The two methods used to treat depression are anti-depressant medication and psychotherapy. Both approaches are equally effective as a treatment and approximately 50–60 percent of patients will achieve remission within 3 months (Clark, 2004).

Psychotherapy

Many studies have demonstrated the effectiveness of psychotherapies such as cognitive behavioural therapy (CBT) or related approaches such as problem-solving therapy for individuals with depression (American Psychiatric Association, 1993). Behavioural therapists work with the individual to undo repeated patterns of negative thoughts, low mood, decreased motivation, and inactivity with the aim of increasing pleasur-able and productive activities and the individual's quality of life. This method of treating depression involves the use of proven techniques that aim to remove depressive symptoms and improve the individual's psychosocial functioning (Clark, 2004).

Depressed patients who receive CBT appear less likely to relapse after treatment is discontinued than patients receiving only anti-depres-sant medication (Fava, et al., 1996). Although there are no large studies suggesting that treatment for depression in patients with diabetes improves medical outcomes, Lustman, et al. (1998b) state that the treat-ments may have this important effect. They found that patients receiving CBT had substantially better HbA1c levels of 9.5 percent (although this is still 3.0 percent above recommended levels to avoid complications in the UK and 2.5 percent higher than advised in the United States) in the six months following the treatment than for patients who did not receive CBT, whose HbA1c was an average of 10.9 percent. In addition, 85 percent of patients treated for a period of 10 weeks with CBT became free of their major depressive disorder, and 70 percent remained free of symptoms at the six-month follow-up study. However, the CBT approach, which is widely used to treat anxiety, depression and problems with social functioning (and is suitable for patients with diabetes), is time-limited in that a course of CBT is usually for less than 16 weeks.

The advantage of psychotherapy over anti-depressant medication is that it has no side-effects when used in the treatment of depression for individuals with diabetes. Cognitive behavioural therapy has been shown to be as effective as medication in treating depression (Fava, et al., 1996; Holton, et al., 1992) and specifically when treating persons with Type 2 diabetes and depression (Lustman, et al., 1996b). When comparing the effects of Cognitive Behavioural Therapy and self-management training, Lustman, et al. (1998a) found that after 10 weeks, remission of depression was 85 percent in patients with Type 2 diabetes treated with a combination of CBT and self-management training, whilst it was only

27 percent in the self-management training group alone. A six-month follow-up found that these rates were 70 percent versus 33.3 percent for the non-CBT group, and that HbA1c was 9.5 percent for the CBT group and 10.9 percent for the control group who received no psychotherapy treatment. This demonstrates the adverse relationship between diabetes and depression, where blood glucose levels remained high during and after CBT, although HBA1c levels were lower than in the control group.

Anti-depressant medication

Studies of diabetes patients being treated for depression with medication have reported absolute increases in remission rates of 17–39 percent (Piette, et al., 2004). This has been confirmed by other studies that have compared patients receiving anti-depressants with patients receiving a placebo (Snow, et al., 2000; Schulberg, et al., 1999). Anti-depressant medication has also been found to be as effective among patients with comorbid medical conditions (conditions that are present simultaneously) as they are among patients with major depression alone (Gill and Hatcher, 2000). The choice of medication is dependent on the range of symptoms the individual presents with, other medical conditions, potential contraindications (drug interactions) between existing medication(s), and any side effects.

Tricyclic anti-depressants are a range of medications, such as Nortriptyline, which have been prescribed for a number of years and have the added advantage of regulating sleep. An unfortunate side-effect of some anti-depressant medications in diabetes is weight gain and adverse cardiovascular effects (Clark, 2004). Newer medications to treat depression are SSRIs (selective serotonin re-uptake inhibitors) such as Fluoxetine which Lustman, et al. (2000b) have suggested is particularly good in the treatment of depression for people with diabetes. These medications have the added advantage that they do not lead to weight gain or sedation. However, SSRIs also come with side effects such as gastrointestinal upset, agitation and sexual dysfunction. Gastrointestinal disturbance may be mistaken as being due to diabetic diahorrea (due to autonomic neuropathy), and sexual dysfunction attributed to diabetes-related impotence.

In addition, the glucose-lowering medication Metformin, routinely prescribed to patients with Type 2 diabetes, is known to cause diahorrea and incontinence as one of its side-effects. Dandona, et al. (1983) have stated that eight percent of the 285 patients with Type 2 diabetes treated with Metformin in their diabetes clinic reported diahorrea. This was not due to autonomic neuropathy which they state is rare. For patients who ceased Metformin treatment in favour of alternative glucose-lowering medication, the diahorrea stopped in 2–5 days. Dandona, et al. (1983) also stated that Metformin is the commonest cause of diahorrea and incontinence among individuals with diabetes.

Because of the lower cost and labour-intensive aspects of anti-depressant medication in primary care, SSRIs such as Bupropion, Mirtazapine and Venlafaxine are used as an initial treatment for patients with diabetes (Williams, et al., 2006; Lustman, et al., 2007; 2006; 1997). Bupropion has been found to be less likely to cause weight gain or sexual dysfunction and does not cause diahorrea. These benefits over other anti-depressant medications may encourage greater tolerance of adopting and maintaining an anti-depressant medication regime (Lustman, et al., 2005). The following comment gives an example of why anti-depressant medication was prescribed but not taken by the patient:

> I was prescribed Amitriptyline by a consultant I was referred to as I have intense back pain. He told me it would also help with my depression. When I read the information leaflet for the tablets I found that they could increase feelings of suicide and anxiety and, on top of that, cause major fluctuations in blood glucose levels. I didn't even bother to take one tablet as I am already depressed enough and have problems with erratic blood glucose levels.

The effective management of depression in individuals with diabetes requires an understanding of both conditions, and any potential contraindications or adverse reactions of medications already taken in conjunction with a new treatment. Older treatments for depression, such as monoamine oxidase inhibitors (MOIs) and tricyclic anti-depressants (TCAs) are more dangerous if an overdose is taken and they have more unpleasant side-effects (such as weight gain and sedation) than newer medications. For these reasons they are used infrequently. TCAs have also been associated with orthostatic hypotension (low blood pressure), urinary retention and heart rhythm defects, therefore making them unsuitable for people with cardiovascular disease and diabetes. Before any anti-depressant medication is prescribed a check of current prescriptive medications that are known to contribute to depression is made. These include some anti-hypertensive drugs (to treat high blood pressure); anti-neoplastic medication (preventing abnormal growth of tissue), and immunosuppressant agents prescribed after organ transplant (Brown, et al., 2003).

Although only considered in patients with severe or life-threatening depression. Electro-convulsive therapy (ECT) is performed on an outpatient basis and provides marked relief from symptoms (Tew, et al., 1999). ECT is known to be safe and effective for people with and without diabetes, having no adverse effects on glycaemic control (Netzel, et al., 2002). Because ECT is suitable for patients with diabetes it provides an alternative treatment option for those with severe depression who suffer side effects from anti-depressant medications or for those where medications are contra-indicated. However, historically in the 1960s, the popularity of using ECT to treat conditions such as schizophrenia had dramatically waned due to the availability of other medication-based treatments to treat the condition, and a strong anti-ECT lobby (Abrams, 1988) of the opinion that human beings should not be subjected to the cruelty of repeated electric shock to the brain, a technique used to slaughter animals, and resulting in the distinct adverse after-effects on the personality and cognitive ability.

Remaining on a treatment regime (recovery dose) for depression despite an improvement in symptoms maintains that status in order to prevent relapse. This has been shown to be effective in patients with depression in extending the depression-free period between episodes with the use of Sertraline anti-depressant medication (Lustman, et al., 2006). Glycaemic control also improved during the depression-free periods. Castaneda, et al. (2002) have suggested that other approaches to the maintenance of depression treatments are being explored which do not affect the individual's weight, physical activity (as this improves insulin sensitivity), glycaemic control and concordance with the medical regime. It is known that exercise is a preventative measure in delaying the transition from pre-diabetes to Type 2 diabetes because of the effect on increasing insulin sensitivity. Wiley and Singh (2003) have also suggested that exercise may be particularly useful in helping to prevent recurrent depression in elderly individuals with diabetes.

TREATING DEPRESSION TO IMPROVE DIABETES CONTROL

HbA1c blood tests determine the level of glucose that has stuck to the red blood cells in the three months prior to the test. When there is hyperglycaemia, the amount of glucose is raised above normal over time (recommended levels being 6.0–6.5 percent in the UK and at or <7.0 percent in the United States). Hyperglycaemia and insulin resistance (the need for more insulin to maintain blood glucose levels) are determinants of the onset and progression of diabetes complications (De Groot, et al., 2001; DCCT, 1993; UKPDS, 1998a; 1998b). As we have already seen, patients are rarely able to meet these targets despite available treatments and good hospital diabetes care. As previously stated, in the UK, the National Service Framework for Diabetes (Standard 3) highlights the need for the impact of psychosocial issues on diabetes self-care to be recognised and addressed. In the United States the American Diabetes Association has cited the treatment of major depression as a way to reduce hyperglycaemia in at risk individuals with diabetes or pre-diabetes (insulin resistance).

Research has taken place to examine the effect of treating depression on glucose levels to assess any reduction and any change in insulin resistance. Lustman, et al. (1997) gave Nortriptyline (an anti-depressant and mild sedative) to depressed and non-depressed individuals to assess any change in HbA1c levels. However, the medication was shown to worsen glycaemic control, although depressive symptoms were reduced in those patients with depression. In a second study Lustman, et al. (2000b) administered Fluoxetine (an anti-depressant medication with fewer sedative effects) to patients with and without diabetes and found that the individuals with diabetes had a reduction in HbA1c levels after 8 weeks of treatment.

A third study by Lustman and Clouse (2005) showed that Bupropion – an anti-depressant medication also used to assist with smoking cessation (Morton and Hall, 1999) reduced symptoms of depression in more than 80 percent of patients with Type 2 diabetes.

Weight loss and depression improvement were also shown to reduce HbA1c levels. As previously mentioned, Lustman, et al. (1998b) studied the effects of Cognitive Behavioural Therapy on the symptoms of depression and its effect on glycaemic control over time. The researchers found no change in HbA1c after 10 weeks of treatment, but after six months of sustained CBT induced behaviour change, HbA1c was found to be slightly reduced.

In terms of treating insulin resistance in non-diabetic individuals with depression, Okamuru, et al. (2000) studied a group of 20 individuals to assess levels of insulin resistance and found that insulin sensitivity was lower than in a control group. Individuals with Type 2 diabetes have a low sensitivity to insulin, meaning that more insulin is required to maintain normal blood glucose levels, termed insulin resistance. This study confirmed that insulin resistance is also linked with the presence of depression in non-diabetic individuals. Because each of the studies cited has shown that glycaemic control is adversely affected by depression it would appear that treating depression effectively with a suitable medication (meaning the avoidance of prescribing Nortriptyline in depressed patients with diabetes) also has the effect of reducing HbA1c. This has proved correct in the treatment of depression in persons with insulin resistance.

Type 2 diabetes may still present in the individual, but this can be delayed if depression-related hyperglycaemia is addressed. More generally, it has been suggested that a recovery from depression is beneficial to all health-related behaviours such as partaking in exercise, undertaking appropriate self-care behaviours for chronic conditions such as diabetes, and relating to the physiology of glucose metabolism (Williams, et al., 2006; Musselman, et al., 2003). The following comment demonstrates this:

> I was told that I was at high risk of developing Type 2 diabetes as I was overweight, had depression, and because I have a family history of diabetes. I had a glucose tolerance test and was found to be insulin resistant. I also had high cholesterol and blood pressure levels. This was like a wake-up call as I didn't want to become diabetic and die like both my parents. My mum was almost blind because of diabetes and my dad lost a leg because of it. I lost a lot of weight and my depression disappeared. I've just had some more blood tests and now my glucose and cholesterol levels are normal, and so is my blood pressure.

The presence and treatment of depression symptoms in patients with diabetes seems to have a varying impact on the individual's ability to reach glucose, lipid, and blood pressure targets set by clinicians. Diabetes patients with depression symptoms are less likely to achieve glucose goals (Karlson and Agardh, 1997), but this improves when they are treated with anti-depressants (Lustman, et al., 2006; 2005, 2000a; Clark, 2004; De Rubeis, et al., 1990). The achievement of lipid goals (cholesterol and high density lipids) does not seem to be affected by the presence of depression symptoms or their treatment (Gary, et al., 2000), although patients with diabetes and depression are known to be less likely to attend tests for blood fats. Rush, et al. (2008) have found that only the systolic rather than the diastolic component of blood pressure testing was better controlled and continued to improve following a course of anti-depressant treatment.

Treating Depression to Prevent Diabetes

It is well known that depression often occurs in patients with diabetes and the condition has been associated with diabetes for more than 300 years (Willis, 1971). The association between depression and diabetes is becoming well recognized, but the chronology of the development of Type 2 diabetes following periods of depression is less well understood (Kessing, et al., 2004; Anderson, et al., 2001). However, in recent times it has become clear that having just one episode of depression doubles the risk of developing Type 2 diabetes (Williams, et al., 2006; Freedland, 2004), with further evidence suggesting that a single episode of depression aged 20–30 years significantly increases the risk of the later development of Type 2 diabetes (Brown, et al., 2005; Weissman, et al., 1996; Spaner, et al., 1994).

This knowledge is substantiated by the evidence that major depressive disorder usually precedes the diagnosis of Type 2 diabetes when the individual is questioned about their medical history (Lustman, et al., 1997). The prevalence of undiagnosed Type 2 diabetes following depression is less easy to calculate due to the milder nature of diabetes symptoms such as increased thirst and frequent urination when compared to the more dramatic presentation of Type 1 diabetes, meaning that it may not be detected for many years. As previously mentioned, Diabetes UK have stated that this period of non-diagnosis may be as long as 12 years before symptoms are recognised during a routine health check or before the individual takes action to visit their doctor (Diabetes UK, 2008).

As we have already seen, depression is associated with prolonged hyperglycemia in the majority of studies of diabetic subjects (Lustman, et al., 2005; 2000a; 1988; Van der Does, et al., 1996). Clinical studies and depression treatment trials have also shown the same association

(Lustman, et al., 2006; 1998b; 1997). The fact that depression is very strongly associated with the onset of Type 2 diabetes is therefore clearly indicated and conversely, those who already have diabetes are at an increased risk of developing depression due to the effects of sustained hyperglycaemia on the body's chemical and hormonal balance. Weissman, et al. (1996) have suggested that having depression increases the risk of developing Type 2 diabetes due to inactivity and weight gain, therefore influencing metabolic changes in the body. It is also the case that many of the medications used to treat depression causes weight gain and sedation, such as tricyclic anti-depressants and selective serotonin reuptake inhibitors, which could also contribute to developing Type 2 diabetes (Brown, et al., 2005).

It is clear that having depression influences decision-making and motivation surrounding all aspects of life, such as dietary behaviour, smoking, exercise, thought processes and participating in self-care activities requiring diligent and ongoing attention, such as diabetes self-management. Research by Ciechanowski, et al., 2003; Lustman and Clouse, 2002; and Lustman, et al., 2000a has shown this to be the case. Almost 23 million people in the United Kingdom (Mainous, et al., 2014) and 57 million American adults have pre-diabetes (Center for Disease Control and Prevention, 2007), placing them at increased risk for developing type 2 diabetes. Pre-diabetes is defined as blood glucose concentrations higher than normal, but lower than established thresholds for diabetes itself (American Diabetes Association, 2012). Whilst not all cases of depression will lead to pre-diabetes, having the condition undoubtedly elevates the risk of later developing Type 2 diabetes significantly. An established link has also been recognised between having depressive episodes when younger (<30 years of age) and the accelerated onset of diabetes in at risk individuals (Brown, et al., 2005).

Even when there is a usual level of self-care for the individual with Type 1 diabetes, depression undoubtedly causes hyperglycaemia that undermines these efforts (Lustman, et al., 2005). The purpose of glucose self-monitoring is to regulate metabolic control, but there are physiological mechanisms in operation to cause hyperglycaemia when depression is also present for which the individual cannot regulate their insulin dosages or glucose-reducing medication. Studies into this area have suggested that depression causes glucocorticoid disruption (the release of hormones such as cortisol in times of stress); an increase in the activity of the sympathetic nervous system (triggering the release of stored glucose from the liver); and alterations in the inflammatory process (Boden and Hoeldtke, 2003; Musselman, et al., 2003; Ramasubbu, 2002) all of which increase the level of glucose in the blood and exacerbate insulin resistance.

Insulin resistance (where the body cannot use insulin effectively) means the same as the term pre-diabetes and is a pre-cursor to the development of Type 2 diabetes. Williams, et al. (2006) and Lustman and Clouse (2002) have suggested that this could be the reason for the development of depression in people with diabetes (including the hyperglycaemia associated with Type 1 diabetes), and the role of depression in accelerating diabetes complications. It has also been found that macrovascular disease (complications of the heart and large blood vessels) occurs without high blood glucose levels in those with depression, having an even greater impact on those who also have diabetes.

Although the link between insulin resistance and developing diabetes still requires further research as it is still only known to be a potential indicator that the condition may occur, there is growing evidence to show that insulin resistance (pre-diabetes) is due to depression. It has been shown for over 25 years that non-diabetic individuals with depression have increased blood glucose levels and a reduced insulin response during glucose tolerance testing (Winkour, et al., 1988; Koslow, et al., 1982). There is strong evidence that individuals with impaired glucose tolerance due to depression later develop Type 2 diabetes (Tiemens, et al., 1996). Furthermore, clinical trials have found that if depression is successfully treated, glycaemic control improves in both diabetic and non-diabetic individuals (Lustman, et al., 2006; 1998; 1997c). It is thought that depression may influence the way cells are affected during the stress response (Williams, et al., 2006; Penninx, et al., 2003; Maes, et al., 1999). This means that the association between depression and hyperglycaemia, and the relationship between depression and insulin resistance could all be related by an underlying genetic factor. There is some evidence to prove that this might be the case. Chiba, et al. (2000) found that certain genetic changes are common to both individuals with insulin resistance who do not have depression and those with depression, but more work in this area is necessary.

Brown, et al. (2005) have suggested that Type 2 diabetes may not be the only chronic medical condition that develops following an episode of depression. However, this is very difficult to measure, although more work in this area could enable preventative strategies to be put in place for these conditions. Brown, et al. (2005) have stated that increased vigilance is of particular importance for young persons who are being treated for depression, suggesting that mental ill-health should be considered as a more important risk factor for future chronic illness than factors such as a family history, a sedentary lifestyle, or body mass index. Similarly Wax (2013) has suggested that the hormones released during a period of stress and depression (cortisol and epinephrine) lower the immune system, reducing the release of serotonin, inducing listless and joyless feelings. Wax suggested that if these hormone levels remain high they can lead to heart disease, hardening of the arteries, Type 2 diabetes, and certain cancers due to impaired immune system function. Chapman, et al. (2005) have also confirmed that depression undoubtedly leads to further chronic health conditions.

Chapter 3

Diabetes and Decision Making

In August 2015 it was announced by the BBC that 3.3 million people now had diabetes of one form or another in the UK (BBC, 2015; Daily Telegraph, 2015a). In the same month the NHS stated that the condition causes 22,000 early deaths (NHS, 2015). By October 2015, the Daily Telegraph reported that cases of Type 2 diabetes had risen by 65 percent since 2005, with almost 3.5 million people in the UK living with the condition according to analysis of GP statistics by the British Heart Foundation (Daily Telegraph, 2015b). These statistics show the rate at which diabetes (predominantly Type 2) is rapidly increasingly, with many more cases still undiagnosed. The impact of such a diagnosis is huge and has far-reaching consequences, affecting every individual in a different way both physically and psychologically. This is shown by the following comments from individuals who were newly diagnosed with the condition:

> When I was first told I had Type 1 diabetes and what that meant I was in total shock and couldn't take it all in for months.

> I couldn't believe what my doctor was telling me – I had to manage this disease for the rest of my life and risk blindness and kidney failure if I didn't.

> You could have knocked me down with a feather when I was told I had Type 2 diabetes. I didn't even feel ill and it was only because of a routine blood test that it was discovered.

It is well known that patients with diabetes mellitus (meaning either Type 1 or Type 2) experience a reduced feeling of psychological wellbeing because of the condition (Stuckey, et al., 2014; Robertson, et al., 2012; Gask, et al., 2011; Rane, et al., 2011; Lloyd, et al., 2005; Anderson, et al., 2002). It is estimated that as many as 50 percent of patients already have a feeling of adverse psychological wellbeing at the time their diabetes is diagnosed (Chew, et al., 2014; Walker, et al., 2012). This is due to the underlying presence of the disease itself creating chemical changes in the body resulting in difficulties in coping with ongoing life events, such as work concerns or family worries which disrupts the individual's daily routine up until when diabetes is eventually diagnosed (Stuckey, et al., 2014; Walker, et al., 2012). Nicolucci, et al. (2013) conducted multi-country research involving over 1,600 participants (patients, family and health professionals). The Diabetes Attitudes, Wishes and Needs second survey (DAWN2) assessed the level of depression as 13.8 percent; diabetes-related distress as 44.6 percent; and perceived quality of life as 12.2 percent.

Having either Type 1 or type 2 diabetes can impact adversely on the individual and their life, not just with regard to disease self-management. Nicolucci, et al. (2013) have reported that 20.5 percent of the individuals in the DAWN2 study stated their diabetes adversely affected their relationship with family and friends; 60.2 percent mentioned that diabetes negatively affected their physical health; and 40.0 percent felt their diabetes medication disrupted their life to the extent that it was a problem. As a result, many of these individuals relied on negative coping strategies [such as smoking or over-eating], with the perception that their diabetes would cause problems in the future (Walker, et al., 2012; Rane, et al., 2011). If the individual suffers from psychological problems that go untreated there is a marked association with poor physical health as a consequence (Bener, et al., 2012); cardiovascular disease (Laake, et al., 2014); and depressive symptoms (Skinner, et al., 2010; Ghiadoni, et al., 2000).

Diabetes, as we have already seen, has been widely reported to be associated with both depressive illness and anxiety disorder which affects health-related decision making. Whilst depression has not been shown by some research to be particularly more prevalent in individuals with diabetes when compared with the rates reported in other chronic illnesses (Kessing, et al., 2003), it is more prevalent among people with diabetes than the general population, affecting around 15–20 percent of patients. Women with type 2 diabetes are twice as likely as men with the condition to suffer with depression (Nichols and Brown, 2003) with body weight being a significant predictor of depressive illness. The presence of chronic diabetes complications such as neuropathy (nerve damage), retinopathy (eye disease), macrovascular complications (heart disease) and sexual dysfunction has also been associated with depressive illness (De Groot, et al., 2001). However, the presence of uncomplicated diabetes without additional chronic (comorbid) health problems appears not to increase the individual's likelihood of developing depression (Pouwer, et al., 2003).

The presence of depression, whether diabetes-related or not, may lead to cognitive decline and can adversely affect the individual's ability to carry out diabetes self-care activities (Sullivan, et al., 2013). The majority of studies examining the condition have focussed on major depressive disorder in diabetes (Park, et al., 2013; Baumeister, et al., 2012). However, psychological symptoms such as anxiety, stress and distress are known to be more prevalent than major depressive disorder (Das-Munshi, et al., 2007; Fechner-Bates, et al., 1994; Coyne, 1994). Additionally, these psychological disorders are associated with increased disability; a likelihood of increasingly declining health; an increased use of healthcare facilities such as hospital appointments for eye and foot clinics; and a greater risk of early death (Goldney, et al., 2004; Callahan, et al., 1994; Fechner-Bates, et al., 1994). Older people with diabetes usually also have other medical conditions that impair cognitive functioning, such as dementia, hypertension and cardiovascular disease. Factors that may further complicate the relationship between cognitive function and diabetes are age, duration of illness, the presence of diabetes complications, and erratic glycaemic control.

The NHS Plan (National Health Service, 2000) states that 'too many patients feel talked about, rather than listened to'. This suggests that many individuals do not feel part of their diabetes team or able to communicate their needs effectively to the health professionals providing their care. It is also the case that they perceive they have little influence over how the NHS works as they are not involved in making treatment decisions. This view has been stated by Munday (1996) and Arnold, et al. (1995) as the reason why people with diabetes should be provided with the opportunity to address the emotional, social, behavioural and psychological, as well as medical challenges that they face. The National Service Framework (NSF) priorities for diabetes care document (Department of Health, 2002) states that 'all individuals with diabetes should be provided with educational and psychological support with the aim of facilitating and supporting self-management'. It is clear from the following examples of patient experience that this is not necessarily the case in practice:

> I have never received any educational materials from my diabetes team – not even a leaflet in the 20 years I've been going to this particular hospital.

> When I last attended my diabetes clinic appointment I told them I'd been diagnosed with depression and that I was taking an anti-depressant [Amitriptyline] that had the side effect of raising blood sugar levels. I've received absolutely no understanding or practical advice to help with this problem whatsoever.

> I don't think my diabetes consultant or nurse have the time to offer information, education or support. My clinic appointments

just involved being weighed, having blood pressure and blood glucose measured, then a quick five minutes with the consultant for him to ask if anything's changed. Then I get told that's it and come back in a year.

The Diabetes UK pamphlet *What Diabetes Care to Expect* (2000) suggests that the individual is responsible for working together with their health-care team as an equal member to achieve the best diabetes management. This implies that the individual is able to communicate in a two-way discussion about their diabetes management and that they can make decisions and ask for what they need. The pamphlet provides a list of members of the diabetes care team which includes a psychologist, along with an ophthalmologist, chiropodist, and dietician. Whilst this is the ideal case in theory, and assumes that this is the norm as it is stated in a patient information pamphlet, in practice there is a distinct lack of available psychological support for people with diabetes (Wilson, 2003a). In a survey of 200 individuals with Type 1 diabetes, only 12 (representing 8 percent of participants) agreed that there was a psychologist or counsellor attached to their diabetes team and that they could be referred to or request a consultation with if needed. Furthermore, 81 people (52 percent) did not know if they could see a psychologist or counsellor is they had diabetes-related mental health issues. Two of the research participants' comments demonstrate this:

> A psychologist or counsellor should be part of the [diabetes] team locally to provide emotional support when necessary. I recently asked for this facility, but was told they don't have that provision. I personally have never received any emotional or social support from my diabetes team. I am not sure if there is such support. I only see the consultant and the nurse and that's the extent of my care team.

> Although I was diagnosed with anxiety and depression by my diabetes team I've had no contact with a psychologist or counsellor. My diabetes care started to suffer because I just didn't see the

point, but I've been left on my own to manage and no one's asked how I'm doing.

The effect of emotions on health

Positive and negative emotions can significantly affect health outcomes, especially the management of diabetes. This negativity impacts both behaviourally and biologically to influence the inflammatory changes which characterise diabetes mellitus (Misra, et al., 2012; Sarwar, et al., 2010). Negative emotions can exaggerate a number of health risks such as heart disease and depression. Stress, anxiety and depression, in turn are related to compromised immune and inflammation responses which are known to exacerbate conditions associated with ageing, such as cardiovascular diseases; osteoporosis (brittle bones); arthritis; Alzheimer's disease; frailty and functional decline; diabetes (Type 1 and Type 2); certain cancers; and tooth and gum disease (Jaremka, et al., 2013; Kiecolt-Glasser, et al., 2002). In addition, negative emotions are thought to contribute to prolonged infections, adversely affecting glycaemic control and delayed wound healing (Kiecolt-Glasser, et al., 2002), particularly a problem for people with diabetes and poor circulation. Immune system disorders such as the skin condition psoriasis, may manifest as a result of negative emotions. Therefore, the association between emotional distress and inflammatory responses is likely to be a two-way process, where the negativity causes the health issue and the presence of that condition causes more negative emotions. This has been described by Jaremka, et al. (2013) as a vicious cycle.

Izard (2009) has stated that emotions play an important central role in consciousness and awareness due to neurobiological and neuropsychological actions that influence thoughts and activities which are expressed in decision making and behaviour. Recent research has shown that, far from being separate functions, emotion and cognition are both interactive and integrated parts of the brain (Pessoa, 2008; Phelps, 2006; Lewis, 2005). This would seem consistent with the high degree of connectivity with the brain's structures and systems (Chew, et al., 2014). As the relationship between emotion and cognition is now well established, it can be seen how emotion directly affects cognition and behaviour when the individual's situation is personally or socially important to them (Izard, 2009; Lewis, 2005).

It is thought that emotions may be either basic (such as anger or fear), which are evolutionary responses; or more complex emotions, such as cognitions, perceptions and beliefs that differ among individuals and cultures (Izard, 2007; Panksepp, 2007). A basic emotional response is a subconscious reaction to an acute situation, whilst more complex emotional responses are processed using perception, intuition and reasoning. Chew, et al., 2014) have stated that experience is a compilation of emotional historical facts as there are no memories without emotions, just as there are no persons without experience; past experience becomes memory due to the emotional content involved. The individual interprets their memories according to the significance of the experience, shaping different meaning for different people according to cognition. Levenson (1999) has suggested that emotions serve as a repository for learned experiences with much variation across individuals, ages, groups and cultures.

A number of human behaviours are shaped by the relationship between cognition and emotion, such as the desire to appropriately self-manage diabetes (regulation). However, behaviour is more complex than being purely emotion-driven, although basic emotion always initiates behavioural action, and thoughts and action in response to more complex emotions (Izard, 2009). This means that the influence of emotions on generating and changing behaviour is dependent on the type of emotion and the situation by which it arose. More complex emotions can therefore effect action via its influence on cognition. Gross (2002) has suggested that thinking thus becomes a key means of guiding and regulating behaviour arising from complex emotions. This is the basis of some diabetes self-care initiatives, whereby the individual feels an action (for example, regular blood glucose monitoring) is appropriate and agrees to undertake it because they are motivated by the perceived benefits and feel they have control. The individual's desire for action is driven by a higher value system determining their health beliefs arising from self-generated values, or derived from a religious-based system (Myers, 2000).

A distinction has been made between cognition and the desire to reach a goal; this process being centred on knowledge, whilst emotion is centred on motivation (Bradley and Lang, 2000). Both knowledge and motivation are usually present in order for the individual's normal social functioning (Scheff, 1983), although intention and activation is not standard and depends on the individual's age and situation (Eisenberg, 2000; Scheff, 1983). Smyth and Arigo (2009) have suggested that both emotion and cognition are necessary in order to attain new life skills and to learn to adapt in a new environment. Brehm (1999) and Kofta, et al. (1998) have stated that because emotions contain energy they inspire motivation to carry out appropriate behaviours. This motivation, driven by emotions, is able to enable speedy adaptation to situational demands by helping the individual to identify relevant and important events and by urging, guiding, and maintaining the behaviours necessary for dealing with these events (Chew, et al., 2014; Levenson, et al., 1999; Kofta, et al., 1998).

If someone becomes angry due to a misfortune, all of their biological systems coordinate so that the individual can deal efficiently with the situation while blocking out all other signals and events. When a stressful situation arises, the thalamus (relay station) signals the brain stem to prepare all major organs and muscles ready for fight or flight. The adrenal glands release the stress hormone cortisol to suppress the immune system to reduce inflammation from any injuries sustained in a fight. Cortisol also stimulates the brain's amygdala (responsible for generating negative emotions) to keep vigilant, producing more cortisol. This has the effect of reducing memory so the hippocampus only provides information about how the individual reacted the last time they had a similar experience. When in a stressful situation, cortisol also stops digestion and the urge to procreate in favour of the situation at hand.

Epinephrine is released to speed up the heartbeat to increase blood supply; the pupils also dilate to let more light in and to allow the individual to be fully aware of any threats, such as pending physical blows, especially if it is dark. If the reality is not a life and death situation these stress hormones act to kill off neurons in the hippocampus (the part of the brain responsible for consolidating memory) creating permanent memory loss. These chemical imbalances lower the immune system, and reduce the release of serotonin, making the individual feel listless and depressed. If these hormonal levels remain high they can lead to heart disease, hardening of the arteries, Type 2 diabetes, and certain types of cancer (Wax, 2013).

Chew, et al. (2014) have stated that emotional systems are designed to conserve energy and mobilize resources to achieve a specific short-term goal. Emotions such as anger are usually short-lived psychological/physiological incidents that efficiently demonstrate the brain's adaptations to the demands of the individual's changing circumstances. Associative memory networks, where past events are stored, become stimulated by emotions to heighten attention and direct certain behaviours forward in the response order. Biological systems are stimulated by emotions to respond, such as the autonomic nervous system to increase, for example, the rate of breathing and blood flow, and the endocrine system to release glucose to the muscles if the individual finds themselves in a fight or flight situation. Further signs of these biological systems in practice include a change in facial expression or tone of voice. It is the case that over a number of years the individual will experience many situations that adapt these responses, serving to give the individual confidence in the environment they have shaped with certain people, situations, possessions, behaviours and beliefs they feel comfortable with whilst avoiding others (Kang and Shaver, 2004).

Brehm (1999) has suggested that the influences affecting the intensity of emotions should be similar to the influences of motivational states. Events that restrict the experience of an emotion can influence its intensity, for example, if a child is taught not to show anger and they repress it, it will eventually boil over in an extreme incident. Research by Brehm (1999) has shown that goal-driven emotional intensity is similar to goal-driven motivational arousal and that both are influenced by the importance of the goal. This can be seen, for example, when something interferes with the expression of an individual's anger and the emotion becomes intensified.

Negative emotions can have a dramatic effect on health because of their effect on cognition and making short-term decisions rather than rationalised long-term choices (Worthy, et al., 2014). When the individual is consciously aware of their cognitions and alters them accordingly (cognitive reappraisal and expressive suppression), this results in improved social adjustment, mental health and general wellbeing (Hu, et al., 2014). Keshavan, et al. (2014) have shown that cognitive training to reappraise negative thoughts is beneficial to patients with schizophrenia, attention deficit hyperactivity disorder (ADHD), and substance abuse disorders in terms of reducing symptoms and improved functioning.

Similar to cognitive reappraisal, a technique known as mindfulness encourages the individual to concentrate on the present and be aware of their breathing and what they can see, smell, feel, and hear rather than to go through life on auto-pilot. This technique can also be used to focus on pain to reduce the discomfort. Research suggests that the brain wanders for around 50 percent of the day, typically lost in negative thoughts about past events, what might have happened differently, or what has already happened. There is a mind-wandering area of the brain, the medial frontal cortex, that focusses on the self. The more practice the individual gains of mindfulness, the denser the anterior cingulated cortex of the brain becomes (the area of the brain responsible for attention, self-awareness and regulation, and monitoring of predictive conflicts such as the distance the individual is from their goals (Wax, 2013). With the use of regular mindfulness training, the individual can also lower their sensitivity to pain. Awareness of anger, and labelling it as such is known to reduce the emotion and calm the amygdala area of the brain so that it produces fewer negative emotions. Mindfulness also activates the 'rest and digest' area of the brain which help regulate emotions (Wax, 2013).

Over time the use of focussed mindfulness techniques has been shown to change the way the individual thinks by shaping the neurons of the brain (neuroplasticity). Neurons (brain cells) can re-wire to overcome harmful thought patterns and behaviour and are capable of changing their configurations throughout the individual's lifetime as a result of their experiences and how they think about them. Thoughts affect the physiology of the brain and, in turn, this physiology affects thought patterns. The brain directs negative information faster than it does positive (Wax, 2013), so when something is recognised as a bad experience, the hippocampus (responsible for consolidating memory) makes sure it is stored and can be conveniently reached for future reference if needed. This negative advance primes the individual for avoidance and fear but, when these emotions are directed inwardly, it can manifest as debilitation and depression (Wax, 2013). This means the individual can be the creator of his or her own stress without any outside influence.

Four sessions of 20-minute mindfulness a day result in reduced pain sensitivity by 57 percent – a greater reduction than drugs such as morphine. Mindfulness is also more effective than relaxation techniques at developing positive attitudes and reducing destructive and ruminative thoughts (Wax, 2013). When the individual notices something for the first time, new neurons grow in the brain; if the individual changes the way they think, new patterns of behaviour are able to then develop (Wax, 2013). Mindfulness-based cognitive therapy (MBCT) suggests that, as with physical pain, depression should not be suppressed. This technique encourages the individual to locate where their feelings and emotions originate in order to lower the intensity. As soon as mindfulness has been practised for a few days the individual will psychologically experience reduced amygdala activity, lessening the feeling of fear, and this will ultimately result physically in a steady heartbeat and normal blood pressure.

Mindfulness lessens physical and emotional pain and makes concentration and focus easier (Wax, 2013). The practice of mindfulness also results in an increased blood flow to the insula and the volume and density of grey matter increases. The insula is the part of the brain that is crucial to understanding what it feels like to be human. It is the starting place of social emotions such as guilt, atonement, moral intuition, empathy, and the individual's emotional response to music (Blakely, 2007). Strengthening the insula enhances introspection which is the key to the practice of mindfulness. Increasing blood flow to the interior cingulated cortex following only 30 minutes of mindfulness strengthens connections to this area, crucial for controlling impulse, awareness and regulation. This explains why mindfulness training is beneficial with self-control and addiction behaviours (Wax, 2013).

Diabetes self-management

Effective diabetes self-management, according to the Cognitive Theory of Self-Regulation, requires the implementation of a positive behaviour and the suppression of an undesirable, competing behaviour (Bandura, 1991). Self-regulation involves factors such as self-discipline, self-reactive influences (sensitivities) and self-gratification (satisfaction) in order to carry out a desired behaviour. The desired behaviour, for example, regular blood glucose testing, must have a certain value to the individual in order for it to generate the individual's increased motivation to carry that behaviour out. When the individual considers the effect of the new behaviour (proactive consideration) or gains approval from others (such as the diabetes nurse), this encourages the individual to continue. The individual may compare the outcome of their behaviour (for example, a reduced HbA1c percentage) to previous personal or social achievements, according to Bandura (1991). This comparison enables meaningfulness to be associated with the behaviour which in turn activates further self-evaluation. Through this repeated process, skills are acquired and the individual develops a sense of self-efficacy (Bandura, 1977b).

Criticism of Bandura's Self-Regulation Theory has suggested that the individual could become overly pleased with their achievements and arrogant with 'self-love' or, at the other end of the scale, become dysfunctional due to misconception, misjudgements of 'self' and prone to depression and destructive behaviours (Chew, et al., 2014; Bandura, 2001; Bandura, 1991). This mechanism of acquiring a sense of achieving self-regulatory behaviour may put the individual's 'internal standards' at odds with 'universal moral standards', thus leading to helplessness and hopelessness (Bandura, 1999a; 1999b). This is very possible for patients with diabetes as, despite proactive self-care, they may not achieve the desired results as the following comments demonstrate:

> I am very motivated to care for my brittle Type 1 diabetes as I have several chronic complications after many years of having the condition. Although I use insulin pump therapy and a continuous glucose monitoring system, I still have diabetes that is very difficult to manage and I've had to content myself with the knowledge that I'm doing all I can, although it isn't enough and my complications have become worse because my HbA1c is higher than it should be.

> My diabetes consultant has told me that my complications [retinopathy and peripheral and autonomic nerve damage] were triggered by several severe bouts of ketoacidosis when I was a young child. Although I've tried my best to manage both the [Type 1] diabetes and the complications over the years, they have progressed and I now find it incredibly hard to keep my diabetes under control.

Self-efficacy

Self-efficacy is the individual's belief that they have the ability to achieve the desired goal of effective diabetes self-management. This concept is based in the theory of self-regulation proposed by Bandura (1991) and is achieved through being motivated to carry out self-monitoring, goal-setting and evaluation behaviours that are carried out despite any barriers that are encountered. A belief in the individual's own ability may therefore motivate them to make particular health choices and persevere when difficulties arise, as can be seen in the following comment:

> I wanted to use a continuous glucose sensor with my insulin pump because I had frequent hypoglycaemia without any warning signs. My diabetes consultant arranged for me to receive the necessary technology and I set about learning how it worked [because the individual was unable to meet with the health educator at the hospital to receive instruction]. When I came to actually insert the glucose sensor into my abdomen, I had problems and, after several attempts, I gave up. A few weeks later I tried again and managed to get it right so it was working and letting me know what my glucose levels were. I think it was the thought of the technology helping me to avoid hypos that forced me to carry on until I succeeded with the glucose monitoring system.

The confidence of this individual to master their diabetes self-management technology arises from learned capability. This is gained via experience where effort is required to adopt the behaviour (Bandura, 1977a). By using varying experiences and by processing efficacy information, learned capability and confidence result. Bandura (1997b) also suggested that the expectation of efficacy is made real by the addition of self-aiding thoughts, values and beliefs which carry the behaviour towards completion. When the individual is unable to make beneficial health decisions however, due for example to depression, the individual's well-being is affected as self-regulation and self-efficacy rely on proactivity and autonomous judgement.

Willpower

Once the individual has decided on an intention, willpower acts to turn the intention into a real behaviour (Baumeister and Tierney, 2012). Similar to mindfulness, willpower requires the individual to exert effort and use self-control when they have to make a choice or encounter temptation. Willpower defers the need for short-term gratification in favour of receiving a long-term return (Duckworth, 2011), such as mustering the willpower to stick to a diabetic diet in order to maintain good glycaemic control. Baumeister and Tierney (2012) have suggested that willpower enables the individual to overcome 'hot' emotional pushes (urges) with 'cool' cognitive ability. Chew, et al. (2014) have interpreted the force of willpower as 'an educated spirit that grows in understanding and has the ability to control emotions'. It has also been described as a trait seen in young children which remains in the individual into adulthood (Hagger, 2013; Moffitt, et al., 2011).

Other research has shown that willpower is associated with increased academic ability in school-age children, greater self-esteem, reduced rates of substance abuse, more financial security and better mental and physical health (Hagger, 2013). However, Baumeister (2003) suggests that the influence of willpower is diminished if it is used repeatedly in a short space of time, resulting in poor self-control when the individual is faced with the next immediate challenge. Research has also suggested that 'willpower failure' is responsible for a number of behaviours that the individual may want to address, such as over-eating, smoking, substance abuse, and shopping addiction (Tsukayama, et al., 2010; Vohs and Faber, 2007). As such, willpower is stronger and more effective when the focus is on just one goal rather than multiple aims (Webb and Sheeran, 2003), such as to incorporate regular exercise into a diabetes self-management routine. Willpower is less likely to be depleted and more likely to be sustained among motivated individuals with a positive mood, attitude and beliefs (Vohs, et al., 2011; Muraven, et al., 2008; Tice, et al., 2007). Chew, et al. (2014) has summarised that positive emotions boost willpower when it is weak, but negative emotions may be supressed by willpower when it is consciously applied according to the situation.

Resilience

Resilience is defined as an individual's ability to maintain their psychological and physical wellbeing when faced with adverse life events by drawing on their self-esteem, self-efficacy, self-mastery and optimism (Rutter, 2012; Yi-Frazier, et al.., 2010; Yi, et al., 2008). These qualities are especially beneficial when applied to diabetes self-management. Depending on the individual's personality, difficult life events are perceived as either stressful, threatening or challenging (Steinhardt, et al., 2009). For the elderly person with Type 2 diabetes, the individual's resilience enables successful social functioning (Mertens, et al., 2012), suggesting that self-reliance is more beneficial to mental health than reliance, social support and material resources. Resilience has also been likened to willpower because, with regular application, it increases over time (Muraven, et al., 1999).

Because health-related misfortune and difficulty 'breeds resilience', it is not surprising that people with diabetes are well-practised at calling on this resource. Experience gained in diabetes self-management over many years of having the condition enables the individual to become strong in this respect, described as the steeling effect (Rutter, 2013; Bradshaw, et al., 2007a; Rutter, 2006) whereby strong layers of resilience are built up. Because it is outwardly visible, it is possible for the diabetes consultant and nurse to objectively view an individual's resilience to a diabetes-related event, such as the diagnosis of a complication, and to assess how that person is coping. Therefore, diabetes healthcare professionals do not have to rely on the individual's subjective assessment of their feelings and the impact of diabetes-related issues. An example of diabetes-related resilience is shown in the following comment:

> I was told I needed some surgery and I was given a date for this. When I arrived at the hospital I was informed that this would not be happening because it had been decided I was too high risk as I had diabetes. I was really surprised to find that this didn't bother me – I was disappointed and felt like I'd been snubbed, but I wasn't angry or depressed. If this had happened 20 years ago it would have plunged me into depression and anxiety and made me ill.

In order for the individual to be resilient they must have resources and reserves to draw from (Chew, et al., 2014). Reserves are formed from the individual's internal strength when faced with difficulty, shown externally as hope, fortitude, optimism, happiness and vitality. They arise from the individual's values and beliefs, shaped by emotional learning, knowledge or religious beliefs (Steinhardt, et al., 2009; Bradshaw, et al., 2007b; Myers, 2000). A lack of resilience therefore manifests as depression, with the individual feeling overwhelmed, disgruntled, apathetic or guilty. Resources are gained from the individual's external support network, such as family, friends, and support groups. Thus, reserves are a stronger resilient factor as they involve more personal characteristics when faced with adversity. This is because adversity hits at a personal level and demands a personal response (Chew, et al., 2014). However, Myers (2000), in common with Bandura (1977a; 1977b) with regard to self-efficacy, has suggested that self-reliance can lead to self-delusion as a result of misconceptions and self-isolation.

The patient's perception of their illness

Leventhal, et al. (1997) have stated that the individual's perception of their illness is a sum of health beliefs and cognitive and emotional representations or understandings. Health behaviours and clinical outcomes, such as treatment adherence, have been associated with these perceptions (Chew, et al., 2014; Weinman and Petrie, 1997). A patient also forms their perceptions about an illness based on how prolonged it is; whether the individual feels they can or cannot take action to improve the illness (having an internal locus of control); how well the treatment works; the patient's understanding of the condition; and the direct and indirect emotional consequences of the illness (symptom experience and worry). In terms of Type 1 diabetes the patient's perception of the condition is continually changing with duration of a disease that currently has no cure, especially if it is very difficult to manage (brittle) Type 1 diabetes and complications have developed. This point is demonstrated by the following comment:

> When I was first diagnosed [with Type 1 diabetes] I just did my injections and forgot about it. I didn't regard it as particularly serious or intrusive, and I wasn't upset or emotional about the

diagnosis. After a few years I developed diabetes-related sight problems, and that's what upset me. I cried and was frustrated, but didn't regard my diabetes as any more serious. When I'd had it for about 25 years I met my husband and he encouraged me to take my health more seriously. I realised why I'd got eye problems and, by that time, neuropathy. I started to see that I had a serious condition and managed it as best I could, but it was too late because autonomic nerve damage was affecting my rate of digestion, making my blood glucose levels very unstable. I now, after 40 years with diabetes, regard my condition(s) as very serious, but it took the complications to make me realise this.

McSharry, et al. (2011) have found that perceptions over duration of diabetes and the patient's understanding of the condition are associated with HbA1c level. This is also demonstrated in the previous comment, and other studies have shown that patients with diabetes are more likely to take on self-management behaviours like regular foot care and increased blood glucose monitoring when they feel they are at risk from complications after a long duration with the condition, and if they already have existing problems (Gale, et al., 2008). Glycaemic control may also be targeted by interventions designed to improve blood glucose levels. Satisfaction with healthcare consultations and provision has been associated with the patient's illness perception and heath beliefs about their condition. Wilson (2003a) found that the meeting of information, education and support needs concerning diabetes care and management was significantly important for patients in terms of satisfaction, as shown by the following comments:

> Because I'm able to ask for whatever I need in terms of information, education or support for managing my [Type 1] diabetes, I am very pleased with my diabetes clinic and the care I receive.

> I recently asked my diabetes nurse about improving blood glucose levels with insulin pump therapy [to tailor insulin dosages to need, rather than two injections a day]. She was so helpful and gave me

leaflets, a phone number for a support organisation, and took the time to explain why my diabetes would be better if I used a pump.

I am very keen to know everything there is to know about diabetes and its complications so I'm always asking questions when I'm at my diabetes clinic. I've been given verbal and written information and health education, and videos and DVDs about certain subjects, and I'm very satisfied with the service I receive.

However, misconceptions regarding an illness have been found to impede efforts by health professionals to assist the patient's understanding of their condition (Donkin, et al., 2006), serving to hinder the patient's self-management efforts (Weinman, et al., 1997). Gale, et al. (2008) found that patients with Type 2 diabetes held a number of beliefs and misconceptions about foot complications 'that differed somewhat from medical evidence'. These beliefs, such as not following medical advice, could lead to the adoption of self-care behaviours that may potentially increase the risk of skin ulceration (Jeffcoate, et al., 2003; Moulik, et al., 2003; Oyibo, et al., 2001). As approximately one in six people with diabetes develop a foot ulcer at some time in their life, and 17 percent of ulcers result in minor or major amputation (Ismail, et al., 2007; Pound, et al., 2005), the need for patient self-care and prevention is significant. However, Gale, et al. (2008) reported that patients failed to carry out a number of foot care behaviours, such as not informing their diabetes or foot care provider of any injury, pain or areas of hard skin; failing to carry out daily foot checks for injury, or keeping the feet well protected. The development of misunderstanding of diabetes self-care activities can be seen in the following quotes from patients:

I always thought that the continuous glucose monitoring system showed real blood glucose levels and I was basing my insulin needs on that. When I mentioned this to my diabetes nurse she told me I was wrong and that it measures plasma glucose, which can be up to 2 points higher or lower than blood glucose. Now I make sure I test my blood glucose if the sensor tells me I am too low or high, just to make sure, and always before I give myself any insulin.

I thought that if I took my diabetes tablets I could eat what I liked as long as it wasn't sweets and cakes. My consultant then told me that things like potatoes and even carrots need to be watched because they contain sugar.

I've always been told not to walk around the house without shoes to protect my feet from injury, but I do walk barefoot or just in slippers because it's a hassle to have to keep putting shoes on.

Coping strategies

Aspinwall and Tedeschi (2010) have suggested that 'future-orientated thinking' or 'proactive coping' is necessary in order for patients to acquire a desired health behaviour. However, this must be desired by the individual and not just by the health professional. Here lies the challenge for health professionals in conferring understanding to patients regarding the importance and reason for self-care behaviours such as foot care and regular blood glucose monitoring. In order for a self-care behaviour to be adopted, the individual must want to do it and recognise the benefit of it. When future thinking/proactive coping is active, the individual is in a state of continual anticipation of any potential difficulties or threats that they may face concerning ceasing the desired behaviour (for example, adopting a calorie-controlled diet and then going on holiday). This then becomes a stressful situation because the individual wants to carry out the behaviour but temptation or difficulties make this more impractical.

By employing proactive coping, the individual will plan a way to overcome this barrier and reinforce their strategy (such as the weight loss diet) to keep their goal possible. Thoolen, et al. (2009) found, in a study of newly-diagnosed patients with Type 1 diabetes, that those with the ability to be proactive were much better able to maintain a long-term (at one year) routine of diet, physical activity and weight loss than those who exhibited self-efficacy behaviour or expressed intentions to do so.

Proactivity rather than future-orientated thinking has been shown to be more easily achieved by the patient when applied to health behaviour (Chew, et al., 2014). However, the individual may require a high degree of support from health professionals and family members in order to achieve a degree of proactivity in their diabetes self-management. Gervey, et al. (2005) have suggested that this is the way the individual acquires the cognitive and emotional agility to succeed. Conversely, patients with the necessary cognitive and emotional support go one step further and feel able to succeed (Gray, et al., 1999). Therefore, patients who can adopt proactive diabetes self-management behaviours and cope well with their condition have a correct illness perception (understanding their diabetes); are able to perceive its position in their life; have self-efficacy; and are able to self-regulate (Chew, et al., 2014).

Looking to the future with diabetes may be overwhelming for some patients, especially if they have poor glycaemic control and/or chronic complications, making coping in the present with the self-manage-ment demands difficult. One of the most difficult challenges of diabetes management is controlling fluctuations in blood glucose levels. This requires a high degree of motivation, tenacity, diligence and anticipa-tion by the patient and the expert knowledge of the diabetes specialist and nurse. Common causes of worsening blood glucose control include infections, surgical procedures, and the use of medications containing glucocorticoids (mainly cortisol and adrenalin, normally released by the body in times of stress). Therefore, both the patient and their consultant should be aware of measures to regain control when glucose rises sharply. Such precautions can help prevent more serious events such as severe hyperglycemia and associated diabetic ketoacidosis (DKA). Diabetes, like other chronic health conditions, can fluctuate in severity, making it harder for the individual to cope at these times. This is shown in the following comments:

> For many years my [Type 1] diabetes control has been very difficult and I've had problems managing it. My consultant tried everything

from testing for coeliac disease to testing for delayed stomach emptying but could find nothing wrong. I then basically stopped trying to control my diabetes because I couldn't cope with the enormity of it all.

I had admissions to hospital for ketoacidosis because my blood sugar shot up and stayed there, no matter what I did. I didn't have an infection, and the problem lasted for about four months. This was made worse every time I had to see my GP or diabetes consultant, as they would remind me that complications were looming. It was like scare tactics but, instead of helping me, I was being blamed. I had no options to control what was going on and I didn't get any help. Eventually everything settled down on its own and I still don't know what the problem was.

I didn't want to think about what I might be like in twenty years. I've always taken things into my own hands rather than let other people help me manage my diabetes. I try to manage it as well as I can day by day and not think about what might happen because it's just too depressing.

These views highlight the need for recognition that coping behaviour is unique to the individual; some patients have unsurmountable diabetes problems; and whilst the patient may cope as best they can this may not match up to the expected goals the patient's healthcare team would assume gives the person the best possible quality of life.

Decision making, diabetes and mental illness

Patients with diabetes experience disproportionately high rates of psychological disorders, as do patients suffering from other serious chronic medical conditions. Psychological disorders can be especially devastating for patients with diabetes. For example, episodes of depression appear to be more frequent and severe than in the general population. In addition, all the most common mental health disorders can interfere with diabetes management. Less active self-care may contribute to elevated blood glucose levels, increasing the risk of acute and long term diabetes complications and significantly lead to a worsened quality of life.

An acute complication of hyperglycaemia is the risk of diabetic ketoacidosis. DKA, as we have already seen, occurs when there is prolonged hyperglycaemia causing the body to break down fats as an alternative source of energy to glucose that cannot be used when there is a lack of insulin, resulting in acid by-products. These by-products, in large quantities, create a medical emergency and the state of acid-imbalance is known to trigger chronic complications, such as retinopathy (Russell, 2012). Ketoacidosis is the major cause of mortality in people with Type 1 diabetes because the condition leads to circulatory collapse, low serum potassium levels and swelling of the brain, known as cerebral oedema (Katsilambros, et al., 2011).

Aliyu (2015) reported the case of an 11-year-old patient with Type 1 diabetes who developed schizophrenia following a severe episode of DKA, becoming unconscious. Associations between Type 2 diabetes and psychotic disorders have also been established, as has the risk of diabetes-related events associated with the use of some anti-psychotic medications (Neuvo, et al., 2011; Baker, et al., 2009; Guo, et al., 2007; Newcomer, 2005), However, the association between Type 1 diabetes and psychosis is rare (Aliyu, 2015). Whilst being treated in hospital for DKA the young patient suddenly developed visual hallucinations, irrational conversation, aggressive behaviour and confused speech and thoughts after regaining consciousness.

The patient had no former history of mental health problems, had not sustained head trauma, and had a normal temperature. DKA was reversed and the patient's blood and urine tests were normal during the psychotic episode. Anti-psychotic medication (chlorpromazine) resulted in a significant improvement. Aliyu (2015) stated that the patient attended follow-up appointments at the hospital and after six months had experienced no recurrence of the symptoms. Acute psychosis of this nature is associated with metabolic, structural neurologic disorders and conditions such as malaria and typhoid, although how this occurs is unknown (Spellman, et al., 2007; Sowunmi, et al., 1993). It is thought that this case arose due to a fluid shift in the brain due to metabolic imbalance brought abought by DKA. Although this is the most likely explanation, glucose, sodium and potassium levels were normal at the time of the psychosis, making it difficult to determine the origin of this episode.

The most common condition affecting adults and children with diabetes is depression associated with poor glycaemic control. It is also the case that frequent and/or prolonged hyperglycaemia results in major diabetic complications; greater healthcare costs; increased functional disability; frequent hospitalisation; and premature mortality (Holt, et al., 2014). However, depression is not purely related to the burden of having diabetes and the necessary self-care requirements that the patient is faced with. Dalsgaard, et al. (2014) have also found that those individuals with psychological distress at the time their diabetes was diagnosed had a 1.7-fold greater risk of cardiovascular complications and a 1.8-fold likelihood of death than diabetes patients without psychological illness. Therefore, physical and psychological changes occur before the diagnosis of diabetes which do damage to the body. As we have seen, Diabetes UK (2008) state that Type 2 diabetes may remain undiagnosed for up to 12 years because the symptoms are mild, but elevated blood glucose levels over this period of time causes damaging to the minor and major blood vessels, meaning that the unrecognised condition presents a significant risk to vascular health.

Diabetes, emotions, and the brain

The function of the brain is modified by a number of significant factors such as education, mood, age, sex, blood flow, and metabolic variations (Cranston, 2005), to name but a few, meaning that function differs across populations and within the individual over time. Recent research has revealed that having diabetes alters the brain both structurally and functionally (Chew, et al., 2014). Changes in the balance of neurochemicals in the regions of the brain controlling affect and cognition have been found to increase the risk of depression in people with either Type 1 or Type 2 diabetes (Lyoo, et al., 2012). However, not all emotional consequences of diabetes result in negative emotions. Many people also report positive experiences reflecting a deepened ability for self-awareness, self-confidence, hope and humour. Enabling the individual to identify with and reflect on good experiences can have immediate and lasting benefits that enable motivation for self-care. However, unfortunately there are also many negative associations with diabetes, resulting in poor self-care and high blood glucose levels.

As we have seen, mindfulness enables neuroplasticity: the growth of new neurons in the brain. However, consistent high blood glucose levels adversely affect the hippocampus region of the brain, impairing neuro-plasticity and increasing mood symptoms (Ho, et al., 2013). Brain studies have shown impairment of neurons in people with diabetes mellitus due to abnormal glucose metabolism, resulting in poor maintenance of memory, learning, and inability to control the expression of emotions (Giacco and Brownlee, 2010).

Laake, et al. (2014) have found inflammatory changes throughout the body of newly- diagnosed adults with Type 2 diabetes who also have depressive symptoms. This particularly demonstrates the effect of negative mood on the immune system and the lining of the intestine [where inflammation manifests as coeliac disease and colitis] (Giacco and Brownlee, 2010). It has been recognised that hyperglycaemia is very damaging to the endothelial cells lining the intestinal tract (Fiorentino, et al., 2013; Naka, et al., 2012). Three factors contribute to triggering the damaging oxidative stress (when cells die or are damaged beyond repair): an abnormal high HbA1c level (the amount of glucose adhering to red blood cells over their 3-month lifespan); the unstable nature of blood glucose levels in diabetes; and the glucose swings from normal to very high incurred before and after meals. This cell destruction is now known to be responsible for vascular complications (Monnier, et al., 2009), and long-term high blood glucose levels cause mitochondrial DNA function to be reduced with perpetual cell breakdown (Hammes, 2003).

This degradation also occurs in other proteins and fats in the body due to high blood glucose levels (Aronson, 2008). Further damage to the vessels of the circulatory system results when the patient has high blood pressure and high levels of damaging blood fats, such as cholesterol, in addition to their diabetes. The breakdown of proteins into glucose (glycosylation) and the oxidation of cholesterol are associated with the worsening of atherosclerosis – fatty deposits inside the arteries (Taguchi, et al., 2007). When the patient has high blood pressure there is a decrease in auto-correction of the microcirculation and the normal lowering of nocturnal blood pressure. This raises the velocity of the pulse, causes miss-coupling of the ventricular blood vessels, and leads to premature stiffening of the abdominal aorta (Fowler, 2008).

The individual's personality comprises their attitude and emotions although these change periodically. Research has shown that rapidly altering emotions over a short time span have adverse health effects, especially on the cardiovascular system because of frequent variations in blood pressure and pulse rate (Bishop, et al., 2001; Lok and Bishop, 1999). A volatile emotional state can also severely disrupt the autonomic nervous system and pituitary/adrenal gland influence on the immune and metabolic systems (Segerstrom and Miller, 2004; Yusuf, et al., 2004; Kiecolt-Glaser, et al., 2002a; 2002b; Ghiadoni, et al., 2000). Conversely, Penckofer, et al. (2012) have suggested that marked fluctuations in blood glucose levels were responsible for anger, depression, and anxiety (those with steeper glucose peaks were more anxious than those with a steady glycaemic rate), significantly affecting health-related quality of life.

A further research trial reported a clear relationship between HbA1c variations at subsequent diabetes clinic appointments and the risk of heart disease in patients with Type 2 diabetes; whilst variability of fasting blood glucose levels was linked to macro- and microvascular complications (Hirakawa, et al., 2014). The marked variation of HbA1c percentage also caused nephropathy (diabetic kidney disease) to worsen more significantly than if HbA1c was usually average, although above recommended levels of 6.0–6.5 percent) at each measurement; average HbA1c being associated more with the development and progression of retinopathy (Penno, et al., 2013). Consistent erratic swings in blood glucose level from high to low and high again may not be recognised in the patient's HbA1c because the lows offset the highs to give an average percentage. This state, however, has been suggested as a predictor of the development and progression of retinopathy, cardiovascular complications, and mortality (Nalysnyk, et al., 2010). Because of the growing evidence suggesting the relationship between frequently high blood glucose levels and oxidative stress to cells, it is concluded that this increases the likelihood of vascular damage and chronic complications of diabetes (Brownlee and Hirch, 2006, Monnier, et al., 2006).

In the same way, erratic variations in blood pressure noted at subsequent diabetes clinic visits were strongly associated with the likelihood of stroke (Rothwell, et al., 2010). For patients whose hypertension was managed with medication, variations in systolic blood pressure were associated with a significant risk of vascular events, such as blocked arteries (Rothwell, et al., 2010). Where there was lasting fluctuation in systolic blood pressure seen at hospital appointments, this was strongly associated with the likelihood of stroke and heart attacks. Where there was variation in the systolic blood pressure of younger patients, this was the strongest predictor of circulatory system complications, but this was not as a result of high cholesterol levels in people with diabetes.

As the brain is reliant on a constant unwavering supply of glucose, it is to be expected that its function can be drastically altered when diabetes changes this fuel supply during hypo- or hyperglycaemia. The extent of these changes has been the subject of research over the past twenty years, although more investigation is necessary. Many cerebral mechanisms are now understood (Klein and Waxman, 2003) and work continues to focus on the impact of molecular changes causing defective cognitive and cerebral function in diabetes.

Improving diabetes self-management

Although the Diabetes Attitudes, Wishes and Needs study (Stuckey, et al., 2014) used psychological and pharmaceutical treatments to target psychological disorders, these types of intervention have not been routinely applied to help patients with psychological conditions to improve their diabetes self-management (Katon, et al., 2010). It is believed that a positive outlook on the self-management of diabetes, resilience and a sense of wellbeing can be gained from the external support of family, friends, health professionals and others with the same condition. It is also thought that screening people with diabetes for depression and offering appropriate management strategies is a feasible option (Hermanns, et al., 2013).

Positive diabetes self-care behaviours and health-related quality of life are strongly associated with positive mental health (Chan, et al., 2009). Several studies have stated that positive emotional health in terms of resilience, wellbeing, gratitude and influence are strongly associated with treatment concordance, exercise and frequent self-monitoring of blood glucose (Jaser, et al., 2014; Robertson, et al., 2013). This leads to improved health outcomes, specifically HbA1c, health status, health-related quality of life, and reduced mortality risk (Roberson, et al., 2013; 2012). Despite this interesting and potentially beneficial area of research, the impact of positive emotional health has been investigated to a lesser degree. The majority of disease management programmes do not address the psychological make-up of the individual, or how this might affect health outcomes. By encompassing both physical and psychological health, appropriate diabetes self-care behaviours, which take time to establish, can be introduced (Forjuoh, et al., 2014; Piette, et al., 2004).

Even fewer studies have looked at the potential effect of positive mental health on blood glucose levels (Skaff, et al., 2009; Ryff, et al., 2006). Those that have been conducted have focussed on poor glycaemic control and depressive symptoms in patients with diabetes and the subsequent negative effect on HbA1c levels (Aitkins, 2012; Fisher, et al., 2010). Although it is already an established fact that negative mood and depression adversely affect blood glucose levels and HbA1c, clinical research trials in this area would be beneficial in providing more information regarding why this is the case. It is thought that several influences may elevate HbA1c such as lifestyle factors relating to the individual's diabetes and self-management demands externally, and distress and depressive illness internally (Golden, et al., 2008).

Chew, et al. (2014) have suggested that psychological interventions involving intra- and inter-personal resources may help to buffer the adverse inflammatory effects of emotional disorders to reduce the risk of heart disease in people with diabetes, or other disease which increase this risk. Learning to value positive perceptions, intuition and reasoning and increasing levels of motivation to embrace a positive lifestyle will ultimately effect diabetes self-management, decision making and quality of life outcomes. It is thought that this is the case due to the undoubtedly positive effect of upbeat emotions on the endocrine and immune systems which are undermined in diabetes (Jaremka, et al., 2013). This in turn fosters self-efficacy, positive behaviours, resilience and health-related quality of life, which feeds back into the loop of improved immune and endocrine function.

The extent of the influence of positive mental health programmes is not currently known without further research. The evidence so far suggests that psychological interventions to enhance positive health would have to be tailored to the individual's needs rather than a non-specific programme attended by a group of patients with either Type 1 or Type 2 diabetes. In this respect, currently available programmes aimed at mental health issues need to become more person-centred. The following comment demonstrates this point:

I had been seeing a Clinical Psychologist for three months after my doctor referred me because I had [Type 1] diabetes-related anxiety and depression. I've had diabetes for many years and basically felt as though health professionals didn't understand my needs as I also have other health conditions. It was suggested that I try and see things from other people's perspectives because I felt that people just didn't listen and were always telling me what they thought I should do. The psychologist then suggested I start attending group sessions rather than the once a week one-to-one appointments I'd been having. I declined because I wanted his time to be devoted to me and my problems, not to have to listen to everyone else's.

As can be seen in this comment, managing diabetes, especially when it is of a long duration and in association with other chronic health issues, can be very demanding for the individual. There is no doubt that diabetes also takes its toll socially, and these issues have been highlighted as important determinants of self-care (Clark and Utz, 2014).

The Stanford Patient Education and Research Centre (2012) and the Department of Health (2005) Structured Patient Education in Diabetes Working Group (of which the author was a member) have stated that the individual's preconceptions and health beliefs may represent a barrier to behavioural change, and that this should be recognised when implementing target interventions. It is also the case that diabetes interventions need to be staged according to the juncture of disease appropriate for the individual; for example, an intervention to encourage self-care in those with long-duration but persistently poorly-controlled diabetes would not be suitable for someone with newly diagnosed diabetes. It is also the case that different groups require a tailored approach to diabetes education, for example, children, adolescents, pregnant mothers, and the elderly (Fisher, et al, 2014). Finally, the psychosocial impact of diabetes must be recognised and included within interventions so that they are not just targeting physical issues. This need is highlighted in the following comments:

> I attended a group that was supposed to help with difficulties patients have with their diabetes. There were a lot of people there, mostly with Type 2, and we all sat and were lectured at. The subject seemed to revolve around blood sugar levels and complications. There was absolutely no mention of how to cope when you feel down and have just had enough of diabetes. Obviously you can't turn your back on it, but it would have been helpful to have this side of things recognised.

> The education interventions I have been on have been very good, but things like moody behaviour and being totally miserable because of diabetes were barely mentioned. In the last session I attended, the instructor just said that it was expected to feel a bit blue sometimes when you have diabetes. I think that's the understatement of the year!

As would be expected, diabetes educators must be trained to deliver intervention programmes and health education that is adaptable, vibrant and culturally appropriate (Stanford Patient Education Research Centre, 2010; Loveman, et al., 1999; Lutfey and Wisher, 1999. The Department of Health (2005) Structured Patient Education in Diabetes Working Group found a number of education gaps where the diabetes needs of certain groups were overlooked, including the need for one-to-one education to be available when necessary; support for children and adolescents with diabetes; insulin pump users; ethnic minorities; carers of people with diabetes and their significant others; and pregnant women. Although the working party delivered their findings to the Department of Health in 2005, stringent cuts to the NHS budget have meant progress is very slow. It is clear that any diabetes-related intervention needs to be appropriate to the patients it intends to reach. This suggests that there must be flexibility, appraisal and re-adjustment on behalf of both health professionals and the healthcare system delivering the intervention (Holt, et al., 2013; Jacob and Serrano-Gil, 2010). Patients would then feel better enabled to make decisions about their diabetes management.

CHAPTER 4

DIABETES AND DISORDERED EATING

Following a diagnosis of Type 1 diabetes, most frequently in younger people, an insulin and diet routine is established to improve glycaemic control. Insulin lays down fat stores and induces hunger and the insulin dosage must be 'fed' with a certain amount of carbohydrates to avoid low blood glucose levels, especially when exercising. This means it is more likely for adolescent females with Type 1 diabetes to have a higher body mass index than those without diabetes (Starkey and Wade, 2010; Domargard et al., 1999). Weight gain is therefore brought about by successful insulin treatment after diagnosis (Larger, 2005). An increase in weight may cause concern and trigger action to halt or reverse this trend, leading to disordered eating. For those with Type 2 diabetes, weight gain will increase the need for insulin or glucose-reducing medication and as a consequence, hunger and dietary intake, meaning that the risk of high and low blood glucose levels are markedly increased (Rezek, 1976).

It is the case that both hypoglycaemia (and the excess insulin in the body causing the hypoglycaemia) stimulate the hypothalamus to increase appetite so that blood glucose levels can be raised to a safe level for the protection of the brain. It has been suggested that the use of insulin pump therapy, or Continuous Subcutaneous Insulin Infusion (CSII) allows young female patients with Type 1 diabetes to take less insulin when compared to those taking multiple daily injections to control their diabetes and avoid hypoglycaemia, potentially leading to disordered eating (Battaglia, et al., 2006). However, the study found no difference in body mass index (BMI) between female adolescents using pump therapy and those taking injections, although insulin dosage per kilogram of bodyweight was lower for those using pump therapy.

Some studies have found that people with diabetes are more likely to have an eating disorder such as anorexia, bulimia, binging, purging, or dangerous dieting habits than members of the general public (Hsu, et al., 2009; Mannucci, et al., 2005; Rodin, et al., 2002; Affenito and Adams, 2001; Watererston, 1995). Neumark-Sztainer, et al. (1996) estimated that adolescents with diabetes may have a 2.4-fold higher risk of developing an eating disorder, and Neilsen, et al. (2002) stated that there is a 15.7-fold increase in mortality of females with diabetes and anorexia nervosa when compared with females with diabetes alone. Other studies have suggested that this is not the case (Herpertz, et al., 1998; Crow, et al., 1998; Engström, et al., 1997). When comparing rates of disordered eating in those with Type 1 diabetes and those with Type 2, no difference was seen (Herpertz, et al., 2001; Herpertz, et al., 1998). Although it was not stated, the reason could be that those with Type 2 diabetes were prescribed insulin to lower their blood glucose, enabling rapid onset of ketoacidosis with high blood glucose levels if dosages were lowered or omitted to achieve rapid weight loss. Further studies which class purging together with insulin omission (as this leads to ketoacidosis, vomiting and dehydration if prolonged) have confirmed this (Affenito and Adams, 2001; Herpertz et al., 2001; Colton, et al., 1999; Crow, et al., 1998).

Deliberate insulin under-dosing or omission is known as diabulimia – attempting weight loss by inducing hyperglycaemia, ketoacidosis and rapid weight loss, and is common in females with diabetes (Shaban, 2013;

Young, et al., 2013). Although a 5-year prospective study found that glycaemic control was unaffected by eating disorders (Colton, et al., 2007), the evidence was unsubstantiated. Conversely an earlier study made a significant link between disordered eating and poor glycaemic control (Engsröm, et al., 1997). This could be due to denial because diabetes is a condition dominated by dietary regulation and portion control, with heavy emphasis on carbohydrate awareness as they are broken down by the body for energy, raising blood glucose levels.

Peraira and Alvarenga (2007) have stated that, in addition to their individual psychiatric predisposition, people with diabetes may be more susceptible to disordered eating behaviours because of the nature of this chronic condition. Jones, et al. (2000) hypothesized that the prevalence of eating disorders in people with diabetes may be explained by patients' feelings of body dissatisfaction, a desire to lose weight because of insulin-related weight gain, feelings of obsession with food, feelings of lost control, the belief that diabetes is controlling their life, and experience of independence or dependence conflicts. However, the reason for disordered eating is highly individual, as the following comments demonstrate:

> I find that I binge eat because I'm unhappy and, of course, my blood glucose levels shoot up. When I'm in that state of mind I don't think, 'Oh, I've had crisps and ice cream and chocolate, so that's so many carbohydrate units. It makes it hard to have the right amount of insulin to cover what I've eaten – I don't know how much I've eaten!

> I began deliberately taking less insulin when I was about twelve because I wanted to lose weight. I remembered that I lost loads when I had ketoacidosis because of an infection and high sugar levels. Unfortunately, now whenever I feel I have to get weight off, say if the diabetes nurse has mentioned that my weight's gone up, the temptation is always there to use that method rather than to eat sensibly.

Research has shown that disordered eating behaviour develops as a result of the individual trying to lose weight (Ackard, et al., 2008) and others have shown that conditions like anorexia are rooted in the individual needing to have control of their lives (Young-Hyman and Davis, 2010). This is an interesting phenomenon as the desire is not to manage diabetes more effectively and have control over it, but to gain control of one's life or situation by restrictive eating and/or bulimia. The individual may also take less insulin due to a fear of hypoglycaemia and a desire to avoid low blood glucose levels – especially when driving (risk aversion) or when working (stigma and a desire not to draw attention to oneself). The motivation for this irrational decision may be that the individual wishes to avoid the unpleasant side effects of hypoglycaemia and the lack of control they have over their own body at these times. This is especially the case if they are reliant on another person to administer something sweet, or a glucagon injection if they fall unconscious with no hypoglycaemic warning signs. A fear of hypoglycaemia can also lead the individual with diabetes to eat more, or reduce their insulin (Cox, et al., 1987). This, in turn, raises blood glucose and may lead to chronic complications of diabetes long-term, as the following comments show:

> When I was in my twenties and thirties I had a responsible job in the medical profession and I couldn't afford to have a hypo at work because I would have lost that job – I didn't even tell my colleagues I was diabetic [Type 1]. As a consequence, I let my blood glucose levels run high to avoid hypos, although I knew I was storing up problems for later. Now I'm in my forties I have diabetic eye disease and nerve damage as a result of prolonged hyperglycaemia.

> Although I've got Type 2, I take insulin. I have the occasional low sugar that makes me feel really shaky and bad-tempered. If I'm going to a social event I don't take my full insulin dose and I eat much more when I'm there because I don't want to feel like that or be like that, especially not with other people around me.

DISORDERED EATING CONDITIONS

The correct diagnosis and treatment of disordered eating conditions and eating disorders among people with diabetes is crucial because these disorders can significantly increase diabetes morbidity and mortality (Peraira and Alvarenga, 2007; Kelly, et al., 2005; Nielsen, et al., 2002) and can also lead to weight gain, poor metabolic control, insulin omission, and an increased prevalence of microvascular complications (Peraira and Alvarenga, 2007; Rydall, et al., 1997). There is a distinction between the terms disordered eating and eating disorders. Eating disorders are psychiatric illnesses marked by disturbed eating behaviours, disordered food intake, disordered eating attitudes, and often inadequate methods of weight control (Peraira and Alvarenga, 2007). Disordered eating includes 'the full spectrum of eating-related problems from simple dieting to clinical eating disorders, such as anorexia nervosa and bulimia nervosa' (American Psychiatric Association, 2006).

Anorexia

Anorexia nervosa is a condition characterised by an absent desire for food and is a severe psychological disorder. It has been classified according to the *Diagnostic and Statistical Manual criteria of Mental Disorders* (DSM-5, American Psychiatric Association, 2013) as a condition where there is an obsessive fear of gaining weight resulting in severe dietary restriction. Anorexia develops more frequently in young women than in the wider population. The majority of studies have focused on young women with Type 1 diabetes between the ages of 15–35 years where there is a higher prevalence of eating disorders (Mannucci, et al., 2005), however Daneman, et al. (2002) states that anorexia nervosa occurring in adolescent girls and young women with Type 1 diabetes is 'extremely rare'. More recent studies have recognised the fact that anorexia also occurs in other populations, such as male patients (Neumark-Sztainer, et al., 2002); minorities (Herpertz, et al., 1998); and people with Type 2 diabetes (Rodin, et al., 2002; Crow, et al., 2000).

A distorted body image is a common motivating factor driving anorexic behaviour as, despite sufferers often being individuals of normal weight or even those who are underweight, they do not recognise this and see themselves as being grossly overweight. As a result, food dominates every aspect of their life and they eat very little, carefully weighing and calorie-counting every morsel so that they are in control of their intake. This mirrors the diabetes lifestyle to a large extent, and it is easy to see how eating little for individuals with Type 1 diabetes means that less insulin has to be taken, gaining a degree of control over both glucose levels and weight. One young woman with both type 1 diabetes and a history of anorexia nervosa described how she took this to extremes:

> I wanted to be in control of my life rather than it being in control of me. I was a normal weight, but portion control and exercise were always drummed into me for my diabetes. I hated it [the condition and the strictness] and started cutting out more and more food until I was basically only eating about 400 calories a day. This meant I hardly needed any insulin, and some days I didn't take any at all because I figured I could live off the glucose my own body couldn't deal with. Eventually I weighed 4 and a half stones (63 pounds) and I was told my heart was damaged. With help from the hospital, this was the kick I needed to realise that I was just slowly killing myself. You cannot have real control over anything in your life, only management to the best level achievable under the circumstances.

An article by Walker, et al. (2002) reported their 12-year follow-up of 14 women with both Type 1 diabetes and anorexia nervosa. The women were aged between 25–46 years with a 26-year average duration of diabetes. Tragically, five of the women died at the average age of 30 years: two were found dead at home having developed severe hypoglycaemia (both women had hypoglycaemia unawareness); one died as a result of deliberate insulin omission and the onset of prolonged ketoacidosis; another died of sudden respiratory arrest two days after bone graft surgery for a non-healing fracture; and the fifth woman died from emaciation following severe autonomic neuropathy affecting the gastrointestinal system, causing intractable diahorrea and vomiting. Each of these deaths was avoidable and the addition of an eating disorder to already volatile Type 1 diabetes was fatal for these women.

Poor glycaemic control over a long period meant that all of the 14 women had developed retinopathy and microalbuminuria (kidney disease) as a direct result. Ten of the women had actually recovered from anorexia nervosa and were of a normal BMI, demonstrating that the damage to their body was irreparable. Both Walker, et al. (2002) and Neilsen, et al. (2002) recorded a mortality rate of 36 percent over 12 years and Walker, et al. (2002) have reported a higher rate of microvascular (small blood vessel disease) morbidity which has also been documented by Crow, et al. (1998) and Rydall, et al. (1997).

In contrast to other mental health conditions, eating disorders have a high prevalence of associated medical complications. Mehler and Brown (2015) have carried out a review of the specific complications associated with anorexia nervosa, stating that the medical complications of anorexia nervosa are a direct result of weight loss and malnutrition. This occurs – as with diabetic ketoacidosis where glucose cannot be used by the cells as fuel – because starvation induces protein and fat catabolism (chemical reactions that break down complex compounds with the release of energy) that leads to shrinkage of the cell and a loss of function. This damage leads to adverse effects on, and atrophy of, the heart, brain, liver, intestines, kidneys, and muscles (Mehler and Brown, 2015). Almost every body system can be adversely affected by this state of ongoing malnutrition (Löwe, et al., 2001). These include physiological complications such as hypotension (low blood pressure), bradycardia (slow heartbeat) and hypothermia (a reduced core body temperature below 35 degrees centigrade).

Medical complications account for more than half of all deaths in patents with anorexia nervosa alone (National Institute for Health and Clinical Excellence, 2004), many being the same or similar to the complications of diabetes caused by prolonged poor glycaemic control. Alternative studies have shown that the death rate for those with anorexia alone is 10–12 times greater than in the general population (Löwe, et al., 2001; Herzog, et al., (1997). The statistics are even greater when the individual has Type 1 diabetes, as we have seen in the studies of Walker, et al. (2002) and Neilsen, et al. (2002). The main risk factors for developing medical complications associated with anorexia nervosa are the degree of weight loss and the duration of the illness (Miller, et al., 2005). The addition of chronic poor glycaemic control (with blood glucose levels >15mmol/L or >270mg/dl) and episodes of diabetic ketoacidosis puts the body under extreme stress, severely altering metabolic parameters.

As weight loss continues due to poor nutrition, individuals with anorexia commonly have dry skin which can split open and bleed, especially on the fingers and toes (Strumia, 2005). This is problematic when there is both anorexia and diabetes present in the same individual. Slow wound-healing associated with poor blood supply and diabetes is well documented. Reduced blood flow and nerve damage (present in 50 percent of people with diabetes) significantly increases the risk of lower limb amputation and ulceration of the feet and lower legs (World Health Organisation, 2011). Anorexic individuals often have cold intolerance and a bluish discoloration of their fingertips, nose and ears (acrocyanosis) due to the concentration of blood flow to vital organs in response to hypothermia.

Similarly, poor blood flow to the extremities is common in people with diabetes due to microvascular damage, the process being amplified by the additional complications of anorexia nervosa (Gobel-Fabri, et al., 2008). Lanugo hair growth (fine downy hair on the sides of the face and along the spine), is commonly seen in patients with anorexia nervosa and may develop so that the body can conserve heat (Mehler and Brown, 2015). Ulcerated areas of skin covering bony prominences such as elbows and heels also develop due to loss of supporting subcutaneous tissue; bruising also often occurs due to reduced subcutaneous tissue (Miller, et al., 2005). Delayed wound healing is a common manifestation of both diabetes and starvation.

When weight falls below approximately 15–20 percent of ideal body weight, there is often the development of gastroparesis (Kamal, et al., 1991). Gastroparesis, which may be severe, is the delayed emptying of the stomach causing bloating, early fullness and rarely, upper quadrant pain. The condition also occurs in people with diabetes (Wilson, 2004a) as it is associated with autonomic nerve damage resulting in slow digestive transit, where patients can experience symptoms of vomiting (relating to the upper gastrointestinal tract), and/or alternating constipation and diahorrea (relating to the lower GI tract). Constipation also often occurs in patients with anorexia nervosa because of slow transit in the colon and because there is very little food available to be processed, resulting in under-activity of the reflex of the colon (Mehler and Brown, 2015). In addition, gastrointestinal disorders such as irritable bowel syndrome are more common in those with anorexia than in the wider population (Porcelli, et al., 1998).

The liver normally produces enzymes (transaminases) to break down and synthesise amino acids and convert them into energy storage molecules. The concentration of the two main enzymes – Alanine Transaminase (ALT) and Aspartate Transaminase (AST) are usually low, but if the liver is damaged, the membrane of the liver cells is more permeable and these enzymes leak out into the bloodstream. The amount of enzymes leakage in almost half of patients with anorexia nervosa is abnormal as weight loss and fasting can lead to mildly elevated levels, although Smith, et al. (2013) have documented severely elevated levels of liver enzymes in adolescent males with anorexia. Marked elevation may be a sign of organ failure in severe anorexia (Di Caprio, et al., 2006).

Mehler and Brown (2015) have stated that liver enzyme levels can also be mildly elevated if the anorexia patient is hospitalised and fed with intravenous dextrose (a form of glucose), a condition known as steatosis, which usually stabilises if the calorie intake from dextrose is reduced temporarily; liver function will improve with nutritional support. When the body is forced into starvation mode the liver shrinks in size and during dextrose infusion, the organ appears fatty during ultrasound scanning, although the exact cause is not known (Harris, et al., 2013).

A further gastrointestinal complication of anorexia nervosa is a condition known as superior mesenteric artery syndrome (SMA) where the duodenum becomes compressed between the aorta and the spine towards the back of the body (posteriorly) and the SMA at the front of the body (anteriorly). Because of the loss of fat (adipose) tissue, this narrows the angle of the blood vessels, trapping the duodenum (Mehler and Brown, 2015). The condition causes pain after eating, a feeling of early fullness, nausea and vomiting. It is also possible that patients with severe anorexia can inhale liquids and solids because of weakness in the pharyngeal muscles as a result of protein malnutrition (Holmes, et al., 2012). As with raised liver enzymes when dextrose is infused, acute pancreatitis can occur where pancreatic enzymes (trypsin, lipase and amylase) are activated and the pancreas becomes inflamed (Morris, et al., 2004).

Acute pancreatitis can also lead to diabetes as the insulin-producing cells of the pancreas are damaged by this inflammation. Anorexia nervosa causes many problems with the endocrine system which affect its function, including elevated cortisol levels that may be associated with the loss of bone density in anorexia nervosa (Lo Sauro, et al., 2008). There are also usually elevated levels of growth hormone (Mehler and Brown, 2015), although levels of insulin-like growth factor are decreased (indicating growth factor resistance) in anorexia patients (Estour, et al., 2010). Anti-diuretic hormone levels can also be low and may rarely lead to diabetes insipidus – a rare condition affecting the pituitary gland characterised by severe thirst and frequent urination that does not contain glucose.

Hypothyroidism is also present in individuals with anorexia where the thyroid hormones thyroxin (T_4) and triiodothyronine (T_3) are low, decreasing in proportion with the degree of weight loss, although thyroid stimulating hormone (TSH) levels are usually normal (Utiger, 1995).

These abnormalities are reversed when there is correct nutrition, but thyroid hormone replacement medication is inadvisable as it can lead to low bone density and ultimately osteoporosis; anorexia also being associated with this complication (Mehler and Brown, 2015).

Not unsurprisingly the severe weight loss and excessive exercise that occur with anorexia nervosa majorly disrupt the generation by the liver of glucose from non-carbohydrate sources such as amino acids, glycerol or lactic acid, enabling the release of glucose into the body, a process known as gluconeogenesis (Wilson, 2014). This results in abnormal glucose metabolism and, in advanced cases of anorexia, hypoglycaemia (Gaudiani, et al., 2012) as there is no stored glucose when blood glucose levels start to fall below normal levels. This can be extremely dangerous as severe hypoglycaemia (<2mmol/L or 36mg/dl) in those with diabetes can lead to death because the brain has insufficient glucose to continue heart and respiratory function (Marks and Richmond, 2007).

Sudden death from hypoglycaemia in those with anorexia is associated with liver failure due to the depletion of glycogen to maintain normal blood glucose levels (Rich, et al., 1990). In contrast with patients who have diabetes and a lack of insulin regulation, insulin levels are reduced by the body in those with anorexia when hypoglycaemia occurs. However, older individuals with anorexia lose this counter-regulation process (Tseng, et al., 2014), and reactive hypoglycaemia [a reduction in blood glucose level due to the body producing too much insulin] has been reported by Yashuhara, et al. (2003) when intravenous feeding occurs. Mehler and Brown (2015) state that Type 1 diabetes sometimes develops in those with anorexia nervosa, although the reason is unclear. Clearly the huge impact anorexia has on glucose metabolism plays a major role, as do complications such as acute pancreatitis which impairs the function of the pancreas. As we have already seen, those with Type 1 diabetes may also develop anorexia, leading to treatment challenges as having both conditions increases the risk of death (Neilsen, et al., 2002).

Mehler and Brown (2015) have stated that hyperglycaemia is only of concern in patients with Type 1 diabetes as it leads to retinopathy and nephropathy. In actual fact, the growing number of individuals who have Type 2 diabetes, especially undiagnosed, is of greater concern due to the epidemic nature of this condition. Whilst Mehler and Brown (2015) were writing in the context of patients with anorexia, eating disorders such as anorexia do rarely occur in people with Type 2 (Herpertz, et al., 2001; Herpertz, et al., 1998) who suggested that there was no difference in the prevalence of eating disorders when comparing individuals with Type 1 and Type 2 diabetes. When patients with Type 1 diabetes are treated for anorexia with structured feeding, a level of 'permissible' hyperglycaemia (a blood glucose level of no higher than 13.9mmol/L or 250mg/dl) is allowed in the shorter term as it is felt that the need for nutrition outweighs the risk of chronic complications of diabetes. Once weight is restored, tight glycaemic control is the aim (Mehler and Brown, 2014).

Further hormonal disruption due to anorexia nervosa is seen in both male and female individuals in respects of sex hormones. Low levels of hypothalamic gonadotrophin releasing hormone (GnTR), pituitary luteinizing hormone (LH), follicle stimulating hormone (FSH), oestrogen and testosterone are seen in patients, affecting fertility, potency and bone density (Mehler and Brown, 2015). In healthy females, the reproductive cycle depends on the release of GnRH which controls the levels of LH and FSH by the pituitary gland, determining menstruation (Tortora and Grabowski, 1993). Female patients with anorexia experience a loss of their menstrual periods (hypothalamic amenorrhea syndrome) as hormonal disruption results in a failure to ovulate, although this state is reversible (known as functional amenorrhea). The lack of menstruation may occur before significant weight loss in 20—25 percent of patients with anorexia, and 50–75 percent experience amenorrhea whilst dieting (Dalle-Grave, et al. (2008).

The hormonal changes associated with anorexia mean that conception is problematic, although the individual may continue to ovulate and can become pregnant despite absent menstruation (Bulik, et al., 2010). As in female patients with diabetes, if pregnancy does occur there is a higher risk of complications throughout pregnancy and for the baby (Koubaa, et al., 2005), and a higher rate of miscarriage (Builk, et al., 1999). Because of hormonal disruption during gestation, 18 percent of pregnant mothers develop gestational diabetes, which occurs in the twentieth week of pregnancy and is similar to Type 2 diabetes with high glucose levels. If the mother already has diabetes, the child is six times more likely to also develop diabetes (World Health Organisation, 2011). With the addition of an eating disorder, developmental problems for the foetus are inevitable.

Disorders of the bone marrow commonly occur in people with extreme weight loss which affect the red and white blood cells and the platelets, with 75 percent of severely anorexic patients being affected (Mehler and Brown, 2015; Sabel, et al., 2013). Anaemia and a low white blood cell count (leukopenia) is seen in around one third of individuals with anorexia, and a low red blood cell count (thrombocytopenia) occurring in ten percent (Sabel, et al., 2013). This may be associated with impaired liver function. Due to starvation, the bone marrow appears gelatinous with a lack of fat (Abella, et al., 2002) because the body has leeched fat, from the bone as a source of energy. Unlike patients with Type 1 diabetes and lowered immune system function, Brown, et al. (2005) have stated that patients with anorexia are not predisposed to infections despite a reduced white cell count.

In common with the brain of a person with Type 1 diabetes who has suffered repeated episodes of unconsciousness due to severe hypogly-caemia (Asvoid, et al., 2010; Bree, et al., 2009; Auer, 2004a; 2004b; Austin and Deary, 1999) MRI brain scans of those with anorexia nervosa have shown brain shrinkage (atrophy) (Ehrlich, et al., 2008). When severe this damage can be indistinguishable from the appearance of Alzheimer's disease on an MRI scan (Kraeft, et al., 2013). Mehler and Brown (2015) reported that weight gain in young individuals with anorexia does not result in restoration of normal brain function as demonstrated on MRI scan, thought to be associated with the duration of the illness as grey and white brain matter damage may be revealed (Lazaro, et al., 2013). Current research using positron emission tomography (PET) scans aims to locate the areas of the brain most affected during starvation in the hope of developing a treatment (Mehler and Brown, 2015). Unlike the long-term effects of high blood glucose levels on the peripheral nerves, damage does not occur in patients with anorexia.

It is known that bone weakness is associated with anorexia nervosa and that 85 percent of women with the condition develop osteoporosis (loss of bone volume) or osteopenia (loss of bone density), with prevalence of fractures being 60 percent higher than the non-anorexic population (Fazeli & Klibanski, 2014). Mehler and Brown (2015) pointed out that bone mass may never be normal if anorexia develops during adolescence as bone accrual continues until the mid-twenties. These individuals have a reduced bone mineral density when compared to women who develop anorexia as adults but also experience amenorrhea (Misra and Klibanski, 2014). However, osteoporosis is also seen in males with anorexia, where it is thought that lower testosterone levels are responsible for the loss of bone mineral density (Behre, et al., 1997) and a study by Mehler, et al. (2008) showed that osteoporosis in males with anorexia tends to be more significant than in females. Osteoporosis is also seen in people with diabetes as they get older as bone health is compromised by the condition. Brown and Sharpless (2004) have stated that it has long been known that those with Type 1 diabetes are at increased risk of bone fractures, especially to the hip, due to osteoporosis and more recently it has been discovered that this also applies to those with Type 2 diabetes.

In the case of anorexia, a low bone mass is caused by reduced bone formation and increased bone reabsorption due to hormonal changes such as the elevated level of growth hormone during starvation. Insulin-like growth factor and growth hormone affect bone metabolism and ensure the maintenance of correct bone mass but, as we have seen, there is a deficiency in those with anorexia (Mehler and Brown, 2015). Similarly, in Type 1 diabetes there is reduced insulin-like growth factor (Jehle, et al., 1998).

It is well-documented that diabetes adversely affects the vascular system, exerting a predisposition towards premature and accelerated disease of the small and large blood vessels. Anorexia also adversely affects cardiac function, causing low blood pressure (hypotension) and a slow sinus rhythm of less than 60 beats per minute (bradycardia) is seen in up to 95 percent of patients (Mehler and Brown, 2015). A low blood pressure and heart rate return to normal with correct nutrition and weight gain (Ulger, et al., 2006). Structural heart abnormalities are also common in anorexia, with pericardial effusion (a collection of fluid in the pericardial sac surrounding the heart) being commonplace in up to 71 percent of patients (Kastner, et al., 2012; Doxc, et al., 2010; Ramacciotti, et al., 2003). It is thought that this may occur in people with anorexia when there is rapid weight loss and low T_3 and insulin-like growth factor levels as the condition is usually reversed with weight gain (Inagaki, et al., 2003), although rarely cases of cardiac tamponade (where the cardiac sac fills with blood and exerts pressure on the heart) have been reported (Kircher, et al., 2012; Polli, et al., 2009).

Additional problems have also been reported, such as decreased ventricular mass, decreased cardiac output, decreased systolic and diastolic dimensions (Kastner, et al., 2012) and mitral valve motion abnormalities (Ramacciotti, et al., 2003). Similar problems to those experienced by patients with anorexia have been reported in patients with diabetes, with pericardial effusion seen in adolescents with Type 1 diabetes (Koronouri, et al., 2009; Hirshberg, et al., 2000). Reduced cardiac output in patients with diabetes has been reported by Pop-Busui (2010) and systolic and diastolic abnormalities by Höke, et al. (2013).

As with diabetes where all body systems are affected by raised blood glucose levels, this is also the case with anorexia as starvation takes its toll. It was once thought that the lungs were unaffected by malnutrition but more recently emphysema, leading to a reduced capacity for oxygen, has been detected in anorexic patients with no other causative factor, such as smoking (Hochlehnert, et al., 2010; Danzer, et al., 2005). Other problems known to occur are pneumothorax (air in the pleural space causing the lung to collapse), and tension pneumothorax (where a valve develops, allowing air into the pleural space which cannot escape, pushing the heart, lungs, trachea, oesophagus and other structures towards the unaffected lung). This is a relatively rare complication of anorexia nervosa but it is a medical emergency (Biffl, et al., 2014; Hochlehnert, et al., 2010). Cases of spontaneous tension pneumothorax and pneumoperineum (air in the abdominal cavity) have developed due to acute gastric rupture via self-induced vomiting in patients who starve and purge themselves (Mehler and Brown, 2015; Morse and Safdar, 2010). Reports of tension pneumothorax have also been documented in patients with Type 1 diabetes and severe ketoacidosis (Steenkamp, et al., 2011).

As we have seen, anorexia nervosa and diabetes mellitus share many similar complications. Ketoacidosis – fat and protein breakdown as an alternative source of fuel for the body – is common to both conditions. In the case of diabetes, glucose cannot be used for fuel in the lack of insulin and with anorexia, insufficient carbohydrates, proteins and fats are consumed so that the body has to break down muscle protein for fuel as an alternative. Both causes of ketoacidosis present extremely serious medical emergencies. Male patients with anorexia are at higher risk from developing ketoacidosis than female patients because they have a lower percentage of body fat and a greater lean muscle mass (Mehler and Brown, 2015).

It is clear that anorexia nervosa is a very distressing and damaging eating disorder. Additionally, males of all ages who suffer from disordered eating perceive and face stigma because anorexia is seen as a condition that only females suffer from, meaning that they may delay seeking treatment (Mehler and Brown, 2015) and may have a greater degree of weight loss with extensive complications when they do finally receive medical attention (Sabel, et al., 2014). Male patients also experience a reduced libido, and reduced testosterone (male sex hormone), luteinising hormone and follicle stimulating hormone levels, and shrunken testes. The totality of complications affecting every body system becomes more severe as weight loss and starvation continue (Mehler and Brown, 2015), although unlike the chronic complications of diabetes which can only be delayed with good glycaemic control, the majority of complications of anorexia can be completely reversed with correct nutrition.

Bulimia

Bulimia and anorexia have both been described as eating disorders in the *Diagnostic and Statistical Manual of Mental Disorders* (DSM-5, 2013) and as disordered eating behaviours (American Psychiatric Association, 2006). Bulimia shares many of the same features as anorexia and some individuals alternate between periods of anorexia and bulimia. The condition is marked by binge eating episodes followed by compensatory purging behaviours (self-induced vomiting and laxative abuse which occurs at least twice a week for a period of three months) and the perception of an abnormal body shape and weight (DSM-5, 2013; Pereira and Alvarenga, 2007). Bulimia nervosa also has two types: purging and non-purging. In the purging type, individuals regularly engage in purging behaviour, including self-induced vomiting or the abuse of laxatives, diuretics, or enemas, whereas in the non-purging type, individuals use non-purging compensatory behaviour to prevent weight gain, such as fasting or excessive exercise (Criego, et al., 2009).

Further eating behaviours affecting people with and without diabetes fall into a broad grouping of disorders that are of clinical significance, but which do not meet the full diagnostic criteria for anorexia nervosa or bulimia nervosa. Criego, et al. (2009) suggest that these include binge eating disorder, variants of bulimia nervosa in which binge eating and purging occur less frequently than twice a week or in which individuals purge after eating normal amounts of food, and variants of anorexia nervosa, for example, in which amenorrhea of three months' duration is not present or in which significant weight loss has occurred but the individual remains above 85 percent of expected weight. There are also milder sub-categories of all of the previous that do not meet full *Diagnostic and Statistical Manual of Mental Disorders* (DSM-5, 2013) criteria, but still may represent a significant health risk. Like full-syndrome eating disorders, these types of disordered eating behaviour also necessitate clinical attention, particularly in individuals with type 1 diabetes where disordered eating tends to persist (Colton, et al., 2007). It is also known that a person may go on to develop anorexia after practising bulimic behaviour (Johnson, 1985) and that clinical bulimia nervosa is prevalent in Type 1 diabetic females (Mannucci et al., 2005; Schwartz, et al., 2000).

With regard to specific behaviours, Neumark-Sztainer, et al. (1996) have suggested that 27 percent of adolescents with type 1 diabetes use purgative practices, and 24 percent restrict their diets in an effort to lose weight. As previously mentioned, the very fact of having diabetes predisposes the individual to a greater risk of developing disordered eating behaviours such as bulimia nervosa because of the necessity for precise meal planning and weighing of food portions, counting of carbohydrate values, the psychosocial issues associated with having diabetes, and the regular self-monitoring of the condition. Peraira and Alvarenga (2007) have stated that diagnosing disordered eating conditions such as anorexia and bulimia in the diabetes population is made far more difficult because of these factors.

It has been estimated that one in every 400 children and adolescents and 11.8 percent of adult men and women has a form of bulimia nervosa and that the condition is more prevalent in women with Type 1 diabetes. Binge-eating disorder, where the individual eats compulsively more than twice a week then purges to get rid of the food, is more prevalent in women with Type 2 diabetes (Centre for Disease Control and Prevention, 2011). As with diabetes, denial of having an eating disorder is common, making studies featuring the patient's experience of dealing with this problem scarce. The National Eating Disorder Association has estimated that 10 million females and one million males in the United States suffer from bulimia or anorexia, and that millions more are struggling to manage binge-eating disorder (Morrison, 2012).

The physical complications faced by those with anorexia are shared by the individuals who practice bulimic behaviour. This is, of course, made worse with the addition of Type 1 diabetes, as the following comment shows:

> I hated the fact that insulin made me fat so I started eating meals properly in front of my parents and then making myself sick a few times after meals. I became hooked on doing this and began to do it more and more. My parents noticed I was getting thinner and took me to the doctor, but I didn't let on because it was my secret. The doctor just suggested I eat more and speak to my diabetes consultant about the weight loss. They didn't realise because I'd had so many episodes of diabetic ketoacidosis because of the bulimia and they thought it was that. I was [bulimic] for many years and now I'm an adult, my teeth are crumbling because I was sick so many times and the stomach acid has eroded them. I also have heart problems as a result, also put down to high blood glucose levels, but I know better. In the end I read in a book that if you put everything you ate in a day into a bucket it would look so horrible, why would you want to throw that up? Although I'm now 30 and I know it was a stupid thing to do, I'm also amazed that no one ever found out what I was hiding.

Fasting

The liver is able to return glucose to the blood when hypoglycaemia occurs; it can also create glucose from energy stores when there is a need, such as during a period of fasting or vigorous exercise. Many people with diabetes fast periodically due to their religious beliefs and not because they suffer from an eating disorder or have a desire to lose weight. However religious fasts seldom exceed 24 hours (Al-Arouj, et al.,

2010). This practice naturally leads to physiological changes as the body attempts to fuel the cells with a reduced amount of available energy.

The transition from the fed state through brief fasting and into prolonged starvation is mediated by a series of complex metabolic, hormonal, and glucoregulatory mechanisms divided into three stages (Felig, 1979): the post-absorptive phase occurring 6–24 hours after beginning the fast; the gluconeogenic phase, from 2–10 days of fasting; and the protein conservation phase, beyond 10 days of fasting. Fasting carries a very high risk for people with type 1 diabetes (Reiter, et al., 2007). This risk is exacerbated in poorly controlled patients and those with limited access to medical care, hypoglycaemic unawareness, unstable glycaemic control, or recurrent hospitalisations. Furthermore, the risk is also very high in patients who are unwilling or unable to monitor their blood glucose levels several times a day (Al-Arouj, et al., 2010).

For patients with type 2 diabetes who are well controlled with diet and exercise alone, the risk associated with fasting is quite low (Uysal, et al., 1998). However, there is still a potential risk of post-prandial (after meal) hyperglycemia when the fast is broken. If the individual takes blood glucose-lowering medication which increases insulin sensitivity, the risk of hypoglycaemia is lower than with medications which increase insulin secretion because with the former, the pancreas is not producing insulin in response to eating. The risk of hypoglycaemia for those taking Metformin to treat their Type 2 diabetes is also low, although dosage may need to be reduced if no food is being taken (Mafauzy, et al., 1990).

The Glitazone group of diabetes medications (pioglitazone and rosiglitazone) are not known to cause hypoglycaemia during fasting, although they can increase the blood glucose lowering effects of sulfonylurea and glinides medication and insulin if taken together (Mafauzy, et al., 1990). Glitazones are known to cause weight gain and increase appetite (Al-Arouj, et al., 2010), making fasting counter-productive if it is for the purpose of weight loss. It is also the case that glitazones require 2–4 weeks to have any substantial blood-glucose lowering effect and therefore cannot be associated with hypoglycaemia during periods of fasting if recently commenced (Retnakaran and Zinman, 2009).

Because there are a number of blood-glucose lowering medications prescribed to suit patient need, it is always advisable to seek medical advice regarding fasting in accordance with the specific tablets taken. A further group of anti-hyperglycaemic drugs are known as sulfonylureas (Chlorpromadine, Glibenclamide, Gliclazide, Gliciazide MR, and Nateglinide) and in this case, it is not advisable to take these if fasting because of the increased likelihood of hypoglycaemia, although if this does occur, it is unlikely to be severe (UK Prospective Diabetes Study – UKPDS, 1998a). However, Chlorpromadine may cause unpredictable and prolonged hypoglycaemia if taken without food (Al-Arouj, et al., 2010), and Glibenclamide (Glyburide) has a higher risk of hypoglycaemia than other sulfonylurea drugs (Schernthaner, et al., 2004; Rendell, 2004)

There is also a group of medications which increase the blood glucose-lowering effect of sulfonylureas, glinides and insulin. These are known as incretin-based therapy (Exenatide, Liraglutide, Dipeptidase-4 inhibitor, Alogliptin, Saxapliptin, Sitagliptin and Vildagliptin). Exenatide has the effect of reducing feelings of hunger to promote weight loss and it does not cause a significant effect on fasting blood glucose levels (Al-Arouj, et al., 2010). Dipeptidase-4 inhibitor is one of the best-tolerated treatments for Type 2 diabetes, although it is less effective at reducing blood glucose levels and studies have suggested that they should be prescribed instead of sulfonylureas; their effects have not been studied during periods of fasting (Drucker, 2010). Glucosidase inhibitor medications such as Acarbose, Miglitol and Voglibose are prescribed to some people with Type 2 diabetes as they slow down the rate at which carbohydrates are absorbed by the body, although they are not associated with an increased risk of hypoglycaemia when fasting as they exert little effect on fasting glucose (Al-Arouj, et al., 2010; Van de Laar, et al., 2005).

Some individuals with Type 2 diabetes are prescribed insulin if their glucose-lowering medication becomes less effective in controlling hyperglycaemia. Short-acting insulins such as Repaglinide and Nateglinide may be used but if the individual is fasting, insulin obviously lowers the blood glucose level and this may lead to hypoglycaemia if no food is taken. For the purpose of fasting for Ramadan, Mafauzy, et al. (1990) have suggested that Repaglinide causes less hypoglycaemia than Glibenclamide. Of all the sulfonylurea medications available, Natenglinide has the shortest working time and is associated with a lower risk of hypoglycaemia when fasting (Al-Arouj, et al., 2010). The incidence of hypoglycaemia whilst fasting for patients with Type 2 diabetes taking insulin is less than for patients with Type 1 diabetes and the aim is to prevent fasting hypogly-caemia as, even when food is not taken, the body produces glucose and these levels must still be controlled. The risk of hypoglycaemia when taking insulin is always present, especially if the individual had been prescribed insulin for a number of years or if they are elderly patients and have a higher risk of hypoglycaemia (Azizi, 2005).

Insulin pump therapy is a medical device mainly used by individuals with Type 1 diabetes (although some with Type 2 also use this method of insulin delivery) that provides continuous subcutaneous insulin infusion (CSII) with a needle placed under the skin. This treatment evolved with the concept that insulin replacement should mimic the physiological action of the body as closely as possible (Fredrickson, 1995). In addition to ensuring a constant insulin supply, the pump user must also learn how to vary the amount of insulin required at different times of the day and night. The level of blood glucose is constantly changing according to physiological factors such as the rate at which food is digested and the type of food eaten; planned and unplanned exercise; stress and emotional upset; and illness (Wilson, 2005).

Theoretically the individual could fast and manage their basal glucose levels (background glucose level without food) with frequent self-moni-toring of blood glucose as pump therapy can be programmed to deliver insulin when needed. With food, a bolus (dosage) of insulin is delivered all in one go, or split over time according to the rate of digestions and type of meal – for example, if it contains a lot of protein but little carbohydrate, this will not raise blood glucose levels as quickly as a high-carbohydrate meal. The pump user determines basal insulin requirements throughout the day and night by monitoring peaks and troughs in glucose levels. Fasting could therefore be undertaken with less risk of hypoglycaemia, but only if insulin and blood glucose levels were correctly calculated.

Diabulimia

Omitting or drastically reducing insulin dosages with the intention of achieving weight loss actually falls under the category of bulimia nervosa (an overwhelming desire to eat a lot of food, followed by induced vomiting and taking quantities of laxatives to avoid weight gain). Diabulimia is a persistent and distressing condition which, because it is largely unrecognised by the medical profession, is referred to in the literature as disordered eating rather than as an eating disorder in its own right in the context of adolescent females with Type 1 diabetes. Eating disorders occur less frequently in young males than they do in young females, calculated at one in every 400 males, compared with 1 in 50 females (NICE, 2004). However, this may be changing. Svenson, et al. (2003) measured the prevalence of eating disorders in young males with Type 1 diabetes when compared with individuals without the condition and found no diagnosable eating disorders in either group although those with Type 1 diabetes had a higher BMI and a higher desire to lose weight. Because eating disorders are less common in young males with Type 1 diabetes than in young females, diabulimia is seen even less often in diabetic males.

Although the problem of diabulimia has been recognised since the 1980s, there is no diabetes-specific measure of the condition making it difficult to assess the prevalence of diabulimia or the psychological effects. Most of the individuals practising diabulimia do not present with symptoms of an eating disorder, so the opportunity may be lost without a high level of suspicion and subsequent questioning for an eating disorder to be picked up in primary care or the endocrinology/diabetology clinician

(Criego, et al., 2009). When both diabetes and disordered eating occur in the same individual, it has often been referred to as diabulimia although this terminology does not properly address all types of disordered eating patterns. As previously mentioned, intentional omission or reduction of insulin dose for the purpose of weight management is included in the DSM-5 (2013) under the category of purging behaviour (Herpertz, et al., 1998). However, this behaviour could be considered an aspect of general non-concordance (Pollock, et al., 1995) or an attempt to reduce hunger, improve feelings of fullness, or reduce the cycle of overeating associated with hypoglycaemia.

Whilst it is difficult to pinpoint the reason someone may deliberately under-dose on their insulin, research does support that the practice is most likely in order to maintain or prevent weight gain (Rodin, et al., 2002; Affenito and Adams, 2001; Crow, et al., 1998). The Diabetes Eating Problems Survey (DEPS), created by Markowitz, et al. (2010), included questions regarding insulin adjustment specifically for the purposes of weight reduction in the context of diabetes care. Validity studies that compare established disordered eating behaviour criteria, interview formats and instruments, versus diabetes-specific questionnaires and interview formats – assessing treatment prescription, adjustment to illness, hunger, fullness, and unexpected outcomes of treatment such as weight gain – are suggested to enhance the accuracy of diagnosis and prevalence of eating disorders and disordered eating behaviour among those with diabetes.

It is problematic to measure rates of diabulimia because this behaviour largely relies on self-reporting by those carrying out the practice. Available figures have shown that this might be as high as 27 percent in terms of meeting the criteria for bulimia nervosa, including binge eating disorder (Young et al., 2013; Smith et al., 2008; NICE, 2004). Fairburn, et al. (1991) and Peveler, et al. (2005; 1992) have suggested that prevalence ranges from 15–37 percent in adults, and Rydall, et al. (1997) state that prevalence is as high as 33 percent in adolescents. In addition to the dangers of inducing diabetic ketoacidosis in order to lose weight, this behaviour has also been found to be accompanied by binge eating, bulimia (inducing vomiting and misuse of laxatives) and excessive exercise – which can induce hyperglycaemia when there is insufficient insulin – by more young females suffering with Type 1 diabetes, shown to be eight percent when compared with one percent of non-diabetic girls (Smith et al., 2008; Colton et al., 2004).

Further research into diabulimia has concentrated on the long-term consequences of this condition at eight and 12-year follow-up intervals (Goebel-Fabri, et al., 2008; Colton et al., 2007; Colton et al., 2004). Inevitably, the under-dosing of insulin and induced hyperglycaemia over several years meant that these young women had developed peripheral neuropathy (nerve damage), a complex condition affecting the feet and hands. Peripheral neuropathy is a chronic complication of diabetes. This condition has two types: diffuse neuropathy, commonly appearing as disorders of sensation in the extremities of the body, and distal polyneuropathy, affecting many nerves of the hands and feet. Goebel-Fabri, et al. (2008) also found that restricting insulin to lose weight increased the incidence (the rate of increase) of death by 3.2 times (Goebel-Fabri et al., 2008).

Although it is not understood why an individual diagnosed with the serious condition of Type 1 diabetes may choose to induce life-threatening complications by restricting their insulin dosages, there are some common factors which make this more likely. As previously reported, Cox, et al. (1987) have suggested that the desire to reduce insulin dosages may also be connected with the fear of severe hypoglycaemia. This experience can be very frightening, where the individual feels that they are unable to control what is happening to them as they must rely on another person when glucose levels are so low that the individual cannot help themselves (Wilson, 2014).

Diabulimia, as we have seen, is far more common in female adolescents wishing to control their weight. This factor has also been linked to the necessary dietary restraints imposed by a diagnosis of Type 1 diabetes: restriction and careful monitoring of the carbohydrate content of food and calculating the correct insulin dosage in order to maintain normal blood glucose levels. Further factors that are known to make insulin-restricting behaviour more likely are weight gain following commencement of insulin treatment for Type 1 diabetes [reversing hyperglycaemia and inducing hunger]; low self-esteem [which accompanies the diagnosis of a chronic disease, marking the adolescent as different from their peers]; and any dysfunction within the family setting [because major adjustments are made to accommodate the high demands of newly-diagnosed Type 1 diabetes into family routine] (Shaban, 2013).

Having Type 1 or Type 2 diabetes requires the sufferer to be highly vigilant about their food intake, including the ingredients that go into bought food and restaurant meals, portion sizes and their carbohydrate value, and evaluating what should and should not be eaten. Diabulimia is therefore a control issue of both body weight and of the condition that imposes these restrictions, although the behaviour has negative consequences. For this reason, diabulimia is usually practised over a period of time rather than being confined to one or two incidences of deliberately restricting insulin dosage. This is confirmed by longitudinal studies showing that diabulimia can become a chronic condition (Goebel-Fabri, 2008; Colton et al., 2007; Colton et al., 2004). A study by Neumark-Sztainer (2002) showed that among women and men with Type 1 diabetes, regular under-dosing with insulin was the most favoured method of weight control.

In an attempt to discover why diabulimia occurs, Markowitz, et al. (2010) conducted a study which asked adolescent females with Type 1 diabetes if they had ever been overweight. The researchers concluded that this was the most likely reason to deliberately restrict insulin dosage and induce hyperglycaemia. Further research by Svenson, et al. (2003) showed that adolescent males with Type 1 diabetes were likely to have a higher

BMI than non-diabetic males, but also found no increased incidence of disordered eating in this group.

Starkey and Wade (2010) and Domargard, et al. (1999) have stated that it is more likely for adolescent females with Type 1 diabetes to have a higher body mass index than those without diabetes. As previously mentioned, this occurs because insulin lays down fat stores, induces hunger; and the insulin dosage must be 'fed' with a certain amount of carbohydrates to avoid low blood glucose levels, especially when exercising. Although adolescents use diabulimia to control their weight gain with insulin treatment, this does not explain why Svenson, et al (2003) found that Type 1 adolescent males were unlikely to have disordered eating, despite also having a higher BMI than their non-diabetic peers. It is clear though that a history of weight problems in the younger female population with Type I diabetes is a strong indicator for omitting insulin to achieve weight control (Olmstead, et al., 2008).

The issue of bodyweight is continually emphasised by health professionals for people with either Type 1 or Type 2 diabetes which can lead to adverse reactions if weight gain or excess weight is perceived as a criticism. This is especially relevant for adolescent females, with low self-esteem who are highly aware of their body image and how others see them. Grylli, et al. (2005) compared adolescent females without eating disorders with young women who had Type 1 diabetes and disordered eating behaviour. The researchers found that the latter had fewer positive attitudes, perceived that they had more problems, had a lower level of self-esteem, and experienced a higher rate of depression. This is demonstrated by the following comment:

> I stopped going to my diabetes clinic because they were always obsessed with my weight – telling me I was overweight and that it wasn't good for my diabetes. The diabetes nurse would weigh me tut-tutting, then the consultant, then my GP, then the Practice Nurse. I feel they don't listen when I try to explain why I'm like this, because my life is a mess. I've now lost 5 stones (70llbs) by

> not eating properly and cutting down on my insulin. I'm going to
> go back to the clinic now I've lost weight, just to show them.

Diabetes health professionals are trained to detect signs of what are termed 'non-concordant diabetes self-care behaviours' so they can determine why a patient might have poor glycaemic control. These signs include the absence of finger-prick marks indicating a lack of regular home blood glucose testing and diabetes self-management behaviour; infrequent orders for insulin or blood glucose testing strips on prescription; weight loss, or fluctuating body weight; erratic HbA1c measurements [venous blood tests showing the amount of glucose sticking to the red blood cells over a three-month period]; changes in mood and depressive behaviour (Ruth-Sahd, et al., 2009). However, for health professionals to recognise any of these changes in the individual it requires someone to know them well enough to notice; a problem if certain health professionals are not visited on a regular basis, and if there is a high turnover of staff.

CONSEQUENCES OF DISORDERED EATING IN DIABETES

Eating disorders that develop in those with Type 1 or Type 2 diabetes each lead to behaviours that have cognitive, emotional and social consequences (Morrison, 2012). Cognitive consequences of disordered eating include: an obsession with food and eating; a disinterest in other activities; a distorted view of food and body image; denial; self-blaming; personalisation; over-generalisation; and poor concentration and decision-making ability. Emotional consequences include: depression and anxiety; irritability; guilt and shame; embarrassment; hopelessness; fear the secret will be discovered; self-disgust after eating; low self-esteem; and feeling that control is lost. There are also social consequences to disordered eating associated with withdrawing from society: isolation; insecurity; mistrust of self and others; and a decreased or absent libido. It may also be the case that some individuals spend a lot of money on binge foods, laxatives and diet pills, or that they shop-lift these items (Morrison, 2012).

Those with diabetes and disordered eating behaviour are more likely to overlook the importance of diabetes self-care, for example, not carrying out regular blood glucose testing throughout the day. If the short-term consequences of poor diabetes control and high blood glucose levels are ignored, ketosis can develop. It is also the case that the long-term implications of prolonged poor control and the development or worsening of chronic complications are disregarded. It is clear that the overall desire to be thin supersedes the pain and discomfort of dehydration and exhaustion and the cognitive impairment associated with poor nutrition. Although anorexia is rare in someone with Type 2 diabetes as it is due in 90 percent of cases to obesity (Daneman, et al., 2002), the individual's diabetes may actually be reversed by restricted eating.

Binge eating without the correct dosage of insulin to cover the amount of food consumed leads to hyperglycaemia and contributes to the development or worsening of complications. Weight gain due to binging is associated with health risks such as hypertension (high blood pressure), hyperlipidaemia (increased blood fats), increased fat stores around the organs, and sleep apnoea – excess fat around the neck which impairs breathing while the individual sleeps and has been associated with the development of Type 2 diabetes due to the effect disrupted sleep has on the immune system (Wax, 2013).

Treatment

As would be expected, treating eating disorders and disordered eating in a person who also has Type 1 or Type 2 diabetes is challenging. It requires a collaborative approach between the individual's diabetes team (consultant endocrinologist/diabetes specialist and diabetes nurse), the hospital dietician (who may also be part of the diabetes team), and a clinical psychologist. These specialists aim to determine the cause of the disordered eating and work together to correct the behaviour. The individual will receive nutrition education, avoiding counting carbohydrate, fat or calories values, as well as learning to recognise health foods as beneficial to their diabetes, thereby moving away from an obsession with this aspect of food and moving towards correcting the eating disorder. They also learn how to monitor their weight normally (Bermudez and Sommer, 2012).

One of the greatest challenges to overcome in treating disordered eating in a person with diabetes is the psychological aspect of the condition. The health professionals involved must be non-judgemental about the individual's health beliefs and behaviour. It may be the case that a clinical psychologist is not available as many diabetes teams across the UK do not have access to psychological support as standard (Wilson, 2004b). A diabetes educator with specialist knowledge of eating disorders may then begin working with the individual (Morrison, 2012). The overall goal of the multi-disciplinary team is to improve metabolic control, and reverse malnutrition and extreme weight loss. It is usual for a parent or spouse of the diabulimic individual to take over insulin administration and blood glucose monitoring, or if they are a pump user, to return to injections (Herrin, 2003), although this clearly conflicts with the individual's feeling of not being in control. Additionally, pump use is usually due to a clinical need because good glycaemic control cannot be attained with injections.

Over time the individual will learn to develop a good relationship with food and not to feel they are a bad person because they have eaten something high in calories. Counselling emphasises that eating a certain food is a choice that is made. Therefore, the individual gradually alters their perception of food. The perception of a person with Type 1 diabetes after beginning this type of counselling is shown in the following comment:

> I felt I'd ruined everything if I had something like cheese as a snack, as it wasn't a proper meal. I often wanted to eat because I was bored or depressed and not because I was hungry. Then I'd eat loads of bad things because I'd already been bad. After time spent with a dietician I began to realise that my binging was not because I was actually hungry. I ate because I felt unhappy, defiant, depressed and hopeless. Eating more meant that I gained weight and ultimately I see this made me more depressed and self-

loathing. I'm now learning to really think about what I eat and why by keeping a food diary.

Eating disorders are therefore psychological diagnoses with physical complications (Morrison, 2012).

CHAPTER 5

DIABETES AND DISABILITY

Living well with diabetes requires good medical care and effective self-management. However, this is not always achievable especially, for example, when fighting an infection (such as flu) where insulin requirements may increase threefold (Jarvis and Rubin, 2003), or when an individual has very difficult to control Type 1 diabetes. Because both Type 1 and Type 2 diabetes lead to continual fluctuations in blood glucose levels the condition exerts very hefty demands on the individual in terms of self-management. Even when blood glucose levels are kept within normal limits as much as possible, the nature of the condition and the impairment in metabolic function often means the onset of complications after a long duration of diabetes (Barnett and Grice, 2011). Good diabetes self-management may therefore only delay or lessen the severity of this eventual onset.

It is also the case that Type 1 diabetes is an auto-immune condition where the immune system, which usually fights infection, attacks its own insulin-producing cells and produces islet cell antibodies (proteins in the blood). These antibodies continue to destroy the insulin-producing beta cells of the pancreas for the rest of the person's life with Type 1 diabetes because this auto-immune destruction, once it has begun, is not reversible. However, because Type 1 diabetes is an auto-immune condition its onset can be temporarily delayed with treatments to reduce auto-immunity, but not indefinitely (Bluestone, et al., 2015). Because of this fault in the immune system it is common that other auto-immune conditions (such as asthma or an under-active thyroid gland) also occur in the same individual, known as comorbid conditions. Conversely, Type 1 diabetes also tends to occur in individuals with other auto-immune diseases (Jarvis and Rubin, 2003). The prevalence of other auto-immune conditions occurring also increases with age due to the length of time the immune system has been dysfunctional (Cataldo and Marino, 2003).

The psychological effects of developing multiple chronic health conditions are not frequently reported as studies tend to concentrate on self-management of a singular condition such as Type 1 diabetes following diagnosis. When subsequent chronic conditions are diagnosed, the burden is on the individual who must go through the further adaptation to their loss of health and learn to develop coping strategies if possible to help them manage and deal with these ongoing problems. In the case of Type 1 diabetes, the patient's Endocrinologist will be familiar with comorbid auto-immune disease, but when the chronic conditions are both psychological and physical, there may be little assistance from or understanding by health professionals who have expertise in one area, but not the others. The following comment demonstrates this:

> I went for a pre-assessment appointment before a steroid injection for chronic pain. They asked what conditions I had and I said Type I diabetes, asthma, under-active thyroid, arthritis and depression. The lead nurse shook her head as if to say, 'We've got a difficult one here'. The assisting nurse kept saying sorry every time she touched me and got in a state when she was trying to take my blood. She couldn't find a vein after five attempts and they called a doctor in to do it. The lead nurse then told me off for having poor veins and for taking up their time. Then I was told the private hospital I was attending was a centre of excellence and that she was a senior nurse with 'years of experience with people like me,' adding that I should remember 'I was only the patient'. Rather than

any understanding I just got a load of baggage from that hospital visit and it comes back to me whenever I have blood taken.

Auto-Immune Disorders Associatd with Diabetes

Coeliac disease

Coeliac disease is a systemic condition (having an effect on the whole body) and does not just affect the digestive tract. It is a chronic auto-immune condition triggered by an intolerance to gluten (a protein found in cereal grains such as wheat that is added to bread to make it rise). Gluten proteins are rich in glutamine and proline residues. Their proline content makes them resistant to gastrointestinal digestion, causing an adverse inflammatory reaction in people who have coeliac disease and gluten intolerance. In a study measuring the reaction to gluten proteins, patients with coeliac disease were found to have an increased Coeliac Disease 4+ T-cell response to several distinct gluten peptides (Solid, et al., 2012). Additionally, patients with coeliac disease make antibodies specific for gluten proteins so that they cannot tolerate them (Lauret and Rodrigo, 2013).

Blood tests taken from coeliac patients typically show low levels of vitamin D due to intestinal malabsorption which may also manifest as the auto-immune skin condition psoriasis. A significantly increased prevalence of other auto-immune diseases has been observed in people with coeliac disease and their first-degree relatives when compared to those without the condition or a family history of the disease (Neuhausen, et al., 2008; Viljamada, et al., 2005; Catalado and Marino, 2003; Vajro, et al., 2003). An early diagnosis of coeliac disease in life and having a family history of auto-immunity are risk factors for developing other auto-immune conditions, while a gluten-free diet has been shown to have a protective effect (Cosnes, et al., 2008). Conversely, a significantly increased prevalence of coeliac disease has been documented in individuals with other auto-immune disorders such as Type 1 diabetes, where 22 percent of patients also had other auto-immune conditions (Triolo, et al., 2011; Stagi, et al., 2005). It is thought that the development of secondary and tertiary auto-immune conditions in addition to coeliac disease occurs because these diseases may share a common pathogenic basis involving genetic susceptibility and/or similar environmental triggers and other undiscovered factors.

Gluten has a dual effect upon the small bowel mucosa. Firstly, small toxic peptides (compounds made from amino acids) induce an innate unspecific immune system response involving the release of a substance known as interleukin which is produced by the cells of the intestinal lining. This promotes the release of a further substance, NF-KB, by the adjacent cells that acts to increase the further production of interleukin and the generation of nitric oxide synthase, promoting oxidative stress (cell breakdown) and helping to prolong the auto-immune response. Interleukin then acts to open the tight junctions between the epithelial cells in the lining of the small bowel. The second adverse effect of gluten on coeliac sufferers is the reaction to this response which causes increased permeability of the cells and initiates the release of immune system peptides. These factors start an antibody reaction responsible for the chronic inflammatory response in the small bowel (Lauret and Rodrigo, 2013).

Ludvigsson, et al. (2007) have described a variety of associated liver disorders that also occur in patients with coeliac disease such as primary biliary cirrhosis (slow, progressive destruction of the bile ducts), auto-immune hepatitis (inflammation of the liver cells due to auto-immune attack), and primary sclerosing cholangitis (inflammation and fibrosis of the bile ducts). The association between liver changes and coeliac disease was first reported by Hagander, et al. in 1977. These findings were subsequently confirmed in several studies showing abnormal liver enzyme levels in over 20 percent of coeliac disease sufferers (Vajro, et al., 2013; Sainsbury, et al., 2011; Bardella, et al., 1995).

Conversely, in patients with unexplained increases in liver enzyme levels, it was estimated that in up to 10 percent of cases such abnormalities were due to coeliac disease (Vajro, et al., 2013; Sainsbury, et al., 2011; Volta, et al., 1998; Bardella, et al., 1995). As with coeliac disease in general, a gluten-free diet is effective in reversing mild liver abnormalities in patients with the condition, although in cases of clinically significant liver disease, dietary treatment alone is not an effective management option (Sainsbury, et al., 2011; Bardella, et al., 1995).

The association between Type 1 diabetes mellitus and coeliac disease has been studied extensively. The diagnosis of the two auto-immune conditions has been found to be often simultaneous or that subsequently coeliac disease develops in patients with Type 1 diabetes (Greco, et al., 2013; Cerutti, et al., 2004). Studies show that the prevalence of coeliac disease among Type 1 patients is between 2.0–11.0 percent (Simsek, et al., 2013; Aggawal, et al., 2012; Salardi, et al., 2008; Mahmud, et al., 2005). This risk is highest when Type 1 diabetes is diagnosed before four years of age. Prevalence of coeliac disease also increases with diabetes duration (Tiberti, et al., 2012; Pham-Short, et al., 2010; Cerutti, et al., 2004).

For this reason, Bakker, et al. (2013a) suggest that children and young adults with Type 1 diabetes should be routinely tested for coeliac disease and because there is a second incidence peak of coeliac disease in Type 1 patients at age 45, the researchers stress that testing for the disease in adults is also necessary. Conversely, the diagnosis of coeliac disease as the primary condition has been associated with an increased risk of developing Type 1 diabetes as a secondary disease in patients below the age of 20 (Ludvigsson, et al., 2006).

For young patients with both Type 1 diabetes and coeliac disease, a gluten-free diet is recommended as it prevents growth disorders due to malnutrition and promotes better glycaemic control via the avoidance of intestinal malabsorption (Camacara, et al., 2012; Abid, et al., 2011; Sponzilli, et al., 2010; Barker, et al., 2005; Bao, et al., 1999). However, more insulin is required as gluten-free foods tend to be higher in carbohydrates. Avoiding

gluten in the diet also has a preventative effect on the development of
vascular complications associated with diabetes (Bakker, et al., 2013b;
Leeds, et al., 2011). It is also known that both Type 1 diabetes and coeliac
disease have a negative effect on bone metabolism (causing osteopenia –
a lack of bone density). Poor bone metabolism increases with duration of
diabetes and/or poor glycaemic control (Lombardini, et al., 2010; Valerio,
et al., 2008), nutritional inadequacies, non-concordance with a gluten-
free diet regime, and the immunoregulatory imbalance associated with
auto-immune conditions (Lauret and Rodrigo, 2013). Unfortunately, the
difficulty in managing both Type 1 diabetes and coeliac disease is not
always recognised by health professionals, as the following comment
shows:

> I've had some horrendous hospital stays for operations where
> having Type 1 diabetes and coeliac disease just seems to throw the
> whole surgical ward into a quandary. On one occasion they didn't
> order a gluten-free or diabetic diet for me and it was easier to get
> my husband to bring food in. They also took away my insulin
> pens and gave me insulin when they felt it was necessary which
> completely upset my glycaemic control. Because I was feeling
> terrible after the surgery I didn't have the strength to argue.
> There also wasn't any speedy assistance when I told a nurse I was
> having a bad hypo, so I ate some sugar from sachets my husband
> had tucked into my dressing gown pocket for emergencies. That
> stay in hospital made me so stressed and anxious because I was
> handing over my care to people who seemed to know nothing
> about my conditions.

Thyroid disorders
This combines with proteins in the thyroid gland to produce thyroxin and
tri-iodothyronine. Both Type 1 diabetes and coeliac disease have been
increasingly diagnosed in patients with auto-immune thyroid disease.
Auto-immune thyroid conditions include hypothyroidism (an under-
secretion of thyroid hormones by the thyroid gland due to auto-immune
destruction); Graves' disease (an over-secretion of thyroid hormone due

to enlargement of the thyroid gland); and Hashimoto's thyroiditis (a condition where auto-immune attack causes under-secretion of thyroid hormone).

The prevalence of thyroid disorders in patients with other auto-immune conditions ranges from 2.0–7.0 percent (Ch'ng, et al., 2005; Ch'ng, et al., 2007; Hadithi, et al., 2007; Spadaccino, et al., 2008). It is estimated that thyroid disease has been diagnosed in 26 percent of patients with coeliac disease and/or Type 1 diabetes; and the risk of developing thyroid disease is thought to be three times more likely because of an existing auto-immune disorder when compared to those without auto-immune disease (Meloni, et al., 2009; Elfstrom, et al., 2008; Ch'ng, et al., 2007; Ansaldi, et al., 2003; Collin, et al., 1994).

The effect of thyroid hormones on glucose metabolism in terms of causing hyperglycaemia is well-recognised (Maxon, et al., 1975). During hyperthyroidism (over-production of thyroid hormones), the increase in thyroxin has a detrimental outcome on insulin by reducing its working time and effectiveness (O'Meara, et al., 1993; Dimitriardis, et al., 1985). This means that patients with both conditions require more insulin to prevent hyperglycaemia if medication is not prescribed to control the excess of thyroxin. Where Graves' disease is undiagnosed, Bech et al. (1996) noted an increase in the level of pro-insulin (the molecule from which insulin is made) prior to meals in people without diabetes. Additionally, untreated hyperthyroidism has been associated with a reduced level of C-peptide (an inactive building block of insulin) to pro-insulin ratio suggesting an association between excess thyroxin and abnormal processing of pro-insulin in those with an over-active thyroid condition (Beer, et al., 1989). The occurrence of hyperglycaemia in association with over-production of thyroid hormones has long been shown to be due to the increase in glucose absorption in the gut (Matty and Seshadri, 1965; Levin and Smyth, 1963).

The body's own production of glucose (in those with and without diabetes) is enhanced in a number of ways when the individual has hyperthyroidism. An excess of thyroid hormones causes an increase in the concentration of glucose in the liver which raises the glucose output from this organ, leading to abnormal glucose metabolism (Mokuno, et al., 1999; Kemp, et al., 1997). A further factor involves an increase in protein synthesis and the mobilisation of fat (lipolysis) associated with increased levels of thyroid hormones. This, in turn, stimulates the generation of glucose from non-carbohydrate sources (known as gluconeogenesis) by the liver.

Vaughan (1967) has suggested that the increased release of free fatty acids could partially be explained by the utilisation of fat induced by excessive thyroid hormones. In addition, hyperthyroidism leads to an over-production of lactate (a salt of lactic acid) that encourages further hepatic gluconeogenesis (Hage, et al., 2011). Hyperthyroidism is also known to cause increased levels of growth hormone; glucagon (making the liver release stored glucose quickly); and catecholamine levels (substances raising blood glucose levels in response to stress), further contributing to impaired glucose tolerance (Tosi, et al., 1996; Miki, et al., 1992; Sestoft, et al., 1991).

There is a fine balance between levels of insulin and thyroid hormones: if thyroxin is over- or under-produced, blood glucose levels are affected because carbohydrate metabolism is compromised. As we have seen, people with Type 1 diabetes may also suffer from hypothyroid or hyper-thyroid conditions in association with auto-immune abnormality. The existence of hyperthyroidism associated thyrotoxicosis (over-production of thyroid hormones) and Type 1 diabetes is known to lead to poor glycaemic control, with increased episodes of diabetic ketoacidosis due to hyperglycaemia (Sola, et al., 2002; Bhattacharyya and Wiles, 1999).

Ketoacidosis, as mentioned previously, is an acute and significant complication of Type 1 diabetes that occurs when the blood glucose level becomes consistently very high (>15mmol/L or >270mg/dl) causing the breakdown of fats and protein as an alternative source of energy to glucose that cannot be easily used in the lack of insulin. This causes extreme and rapid weight loss, being the basis of high-protein diets, and is worryingly sometimes induced by those individuals prescribed insulin for Type 1 diabetes by omitting insulin dosage to deliberately cause hyperglycaemia. Predominantly in people with Type 1 diabetes, (although people with Type 2 diabetes may also need to take insulin and may suffer from this condition), ketoacidosis is frequently seen due to forgetting to inject insulin or under-dosing when insulin requirements increase during illness or stress.

The under-production of thyroid hormones in hypothyroidism also affects blood glucose levels. The liver has been found to produce less glucose in patients with Type 1 diabetes and hypothyroidism meaning that less insulin is required (Okajima and Ui, 1979). This suggests that less insulin is necessary because blood glucose does not rise in the same way as in a person with Type 1 diabetes without an under-active thyroid gland. However, when thyroid function is normalised with thyroxin medication, this may lead to higher blood glucose levels and adverse effects on glycaemic control if insulin dosages are not increased to accommodate this.

Frequent and unexplained hypoglycaemia in patients with Type 1 diabetes may suggest the development of hypothyroidism and this situation is reversed with the commencement of thyroxin medication (Leong, et al., 1999). Other studies however have shown that hypothyroidism has no effect on the activity of insulin (Maratou, et al., 2009; Dimitriardis, et al., 2006; Cettour-Rose, et al., 2005). Frequent hypoglycaemia in Type 1 diabetes and associated hypothyroidism is thought to be due to an alteration in the way body tissues use glucose rather than because of reduced thyroid hormones (Lai, et al., 2011; Rochon, et al., 2003; Dimitriardis, et al., 1997). However, from the author's experience, undiagnosed hypothyroidism can also cause dramatic swings in blood glucose levels between hypo- and hyperglycaemia in brittle (difficult to control) Type 1 diabetes. A link has been found between increased levels of thyroid stimulating hormone (TSH) resulting in hypothyroidism, and the development of metabolic syndrome: biochemical and physical abnormalities associated with the development of cardiovascular disease and Type 2 diabetes (Erdogan, et al., 2011; Lai, et al., 2011).

Although the previously-discussed thyroid conditions are in relation to auto-immune attack and their association with Type 1 diabetes, Chen, et al. (2007) have found an increased risk of neuropathy (nerve damage) in patients with an under-active thyroid and Type 2 diabetes. This finding (contrary to the understanding that low levels of thyroid hormone are associated with hypoglycaemia) assumes an increase in blood glucose levels in association with low levels of thyroid hormone. Neuropathy may occur because Type 2 diabetes develops as a result of metabolic syndrome and adverse changes to the metabolism (controlled by thyroid hormones), potentially explaining the hyperglycaemia.

As with undiagnosed Type 2 diabetes where heart disease develops due to prolonged hyperglycaemia (Diabetes UK, 2008), there may also be a connection with unsynchronised insulin and thyroid hormone levels in Type 2 diabetes, although it is not an auto-immune condition like Type 1. In terms of diabetic nephropathy (kidney damage), renal function in patients with treated under-active thyroid disease has been found to improve (Den Hollander, et al., 2005; Singer, et al., 2001), although diabetic retinopathy (eye disease) appeared to worsen with the condition (Yang, et al., 2010). The presence of untreated hypothyroidism is therefore a risk factor for the development or worsening of heart disease and retinopathy in patients with Type 2 diabetes. It is also the case that when the blood vessels of the eye are compromised in diabetes this makes the optic nerve more susceptible to the pressure exerted by the enlargement of the extraocular muscles. This increases the incidence of a condition known as dysthyroid optic neuropathy in patients with diabetes and an over-active thyroid due to changes to the eye in Graves' disease (Kalmann and Mourits, 1999).

Further evidence of the adverse relationship between a reduced level of thyroid hormones and insulin has been shown by Coiro, et al. (1997)

where individuals with Type 1 diabetes and good glycaemic control had low overnight levels of thyroid stimulating hormone rather than the usual peak, suggesting metabolic changes incurred with Type 1 also alter the control of TSH. Furthermore, if a patient has Graves' disease (an over-production of thyroid hormones) there is a higher risk of developing Type 1 diabetes. It is also known that where the pancreas produces more insulin in pre-diabetes (or untreated Type 2 diabetes) in an attempt to lower blood glucose levels to normal, the presence of this excess insulin increases the size of the thyroid gland causing nodules to appear (Ayturk, et al., 2009; Rezzonico, et al., 2008).

The experience of one individual with long-duration Type 1 diabetes who then developed hypothyroidism is documented in the following comment:

> I'd had diabetes for 25 years when I was told I also had an under-active thyroid after routine blood tests. I'd been tired and had no energy for a long time and my brain seemed very slow. I was started on a low dose of thyroxin but didn't feel any different, with blood tests every three months, and was told each time that the condition was getting worse. My blood sugars were up and down without explanation. My diabetes consultant said I wasn't looking after myself properly and warned that my mild sight problems would get more serious if I didn't do more to help myself. I felt it wasn't my fault and read up on low thyroid and told the doctor that it could cause high blood sugars, but he disagreed with me that my thyroid was the problem, which was frustrating.

Although a gluten-free diet is beneficial to the management of coeliac disease, autoimmune thyroid conditions have still been diagnosed in patients, suggesting that the reduced antibody and inflammatory response achieved by the restriction of gluten in the diet does not convey protection to the thyroid gland in the same respect that it alleviates the adverse effects of coeliac disease. This has been demonstrated by several studies (Metso, et al., 2012; Mainardi, et al., 2002). Other studies however have shown that thyroid antibodies are decreased after two to three years of sustaining a gluten-free diet (Ventura, et al., 2000), and the normalisation of thyroid function after one year of adopting a gluten-free diet has been shown by Sategna-Guidetti, et al. (2001). However, Diamanti, et al. (2011) have suggested that the difference in outcomes may be due to the patient's duration of eating a gluten-free diet.

The association between Type 1 diabetes and auto-immune thyroid conditions is clear and this relationship has adverse implications in respect of impaired growth and development in young patients, as well as negative effects on growth and cell metabolism. As with other chronic health conditions, early detection of both Type 1 diabetes and auto-immune thyroid disorders enables treatment and maintenance of the disease to delay or ameliorate further complications.

Addison's disease
The two adrenal glands lie on top of the kidneys. The outer layers (adrenal cortex) secrete a complex variety of hormones: the mineralcorticoids such as aldosterone (increasing the uptake of sodium and increasing the secretion of potassium); and the glucocorticoids, such as hydrocortisone, known as cortisol; and androgens, known as sex hormones (Prime, 1987). Addison's disease (also known as chronic cortical hypofunction or adrenocortical insufficiency) develops due to slow destruction of the adrenal cortex due to auto-immune mechanism.

The condition may take many years to develop and may only be obvious in the middle-aged when the patient develops increased skin pigmentation due to a lack of corticosteroids. Other indicators of Addison's disease include a greater amount of sodium being lost in the urine with an associated rise in levels of blood potassium; and hypoglycaemia (Prime, 1987). The latter is, of course, most frequently associated with Type 1 diabetes when there is an excess of insulin injected by the patient or when a meal is delayed. However, people with Type 2 diabetes may also experience hypoglycaemia if blood glucose lowering medication is taken without food or if prolonged physical exercise has been undertaken, reducing blood glucose levels further. Treatment of Addison's disease is by replacement of corticosteroids in the form of hydrocortisone which may have to be taken for a long duration. There is also a more severe form of this condition known as acute adrenocortical hypofunction (also called Addison's crisis or adrenal crisis) which is a medical emergency. It occurs due to a sudden reduction in hydrocortisone because the patient has an infection or because they omit to take their steroid therapy. The individual loses consciousness, requiring rapid intravenous infusion of hydrocortisone (Prime, 1987).

Addison's disease is rare and, in the UK, incidence is only five cases per million of the population per year (Kong and Jevcoate, 1994) with a prevalence of 110 per million; however, it is five times more common in people with Type 1 diabetes as it is a related auto-immune condition (MacCuish and Irvine, 1975). It may be difficult to diagnose the presence of Addison's disease because it often presents with non-specific features that are of slow onset. Studies show that between 10–18 percent of patients with Type 1 diabetes will go on to develop Addison's disease as it is more common in this group than in the general population (Nerup, 1974, Irvine and Barnes, 1972). Conversely however, the occurrence of Type 1 diabetes in those with Addison' disease is much lower at only 1.2 percent (Zelissenet, et al., 1995). Type 1 diabetes therefore precedes the development of adrenocortical insufficiency in the majority of patients.

McAuley and Frier (1999) reported the case of a 19-year old man with Type 1 diabetes and auto-immune hypothyroidism. He began to experience frequent and unexplained severe hypoglycaemia (disabling low blood glucose levels requiring the assistance of another person) over several months despite reducing his insulin dosage considerably. His recurrent hypoglycaemia was discovered to be due to adrenal insufficiency (reduced hormone production due to auto-immune damage, decreasing hormones such as cortisol which maintains the levels of glucose in blood plasma). This case study demonstrated that undiagnosed Addison's disease can cause severe hypoglycaemia due to its influence on glycaemic control.

Furthermore, if there is an overall reduction by the patient in insulin requirement (corresponding with continual low glucose readings) by 15–20 percent, underlying Addison's disease is indicated. There is also abnormal skin pigmentation and a lack of growth in young and adolescent patients, suggesting that investigation of these symptoms should also involve thyroid function tests as Addison's disease, thyroid dysfunction and Type 1 diabetes are closely associated auto-immune conditions.

It has been reported that patients with Addison's disease are also at-risk of developing coeliac disease as this is a further auto-immune condition (Myhre, et al., 2013; O'Leary, et al., 2002; Heneghan, et al., 1997; Reunala, et al., 1987). Several studies have shown a 5.0–12 percent prevalence of coeliac disease in patients with pre-existing Addison's disease (Myhre, et al., 2013; Betterle, et al., 2006; Biagi, et al., 2006; O'Leary, et al., 2002). Conversely, this is also confirmed, demonstrating an increased risk of developing Addison's disease among coeliac disease patients (Elfstrom, et al., 2007). Whilst being a vital component in the management of coeliac disease, adopting a gluten-free diet does not alter the natural history of Addison's disease (Betterle, et al., 2006), therefore it does not offer any preventative value or protection from the slow onset of this secondary auto-immune condition.

Asthma
Asthma is a condition characterised by breathlessness due to generalised narrowing of the airways throughout the lungs. There are two different types of asthma in terms of the cause: extrinisic, where external factors (allergens) such as smoke, pollen, dust etc. trigger an attack, and intrinsic, where there is no apparent external cause. Asthma can be episodic, where attacks occur at any time for a variable length and severity; chronic, where the patient has a persistent wheeze and cough and is permanently breathless with frequent chest infections; and status asthmaticus, where

the attack is severe and lasts for more than 24 hours with no response to medication, leading to an increased heart rate and potential loss of conciseness (Prime, 1987).

A progressive increase in the prevalence of Type 1 diabetes and asthma has been noted among populations in developed countries (Hsia, et al., 2015) and an increase in auto-immune diseases as a whole (Benchimol, et al., 2015). This could potentially be due to the nature of these chronic health issues and their treatments. Supporting the findings of a recent increase in prevalence of the two conditions by Hsia, et al. (2015), a European study had previously demonstrated that the risk of asthma is significantly decreased in children with Type 1 diabetes (The Eurodiab Ace Study Group and the Eurodiab Ace Substudy 2 Study Group, 1998).There is undoubtedly a negative association between asthma symptoms and Type 1 diabetes, and it has been shown that non-diabetic siblings are exposed to the protective effect of a stronger immune system due to environmental factors encountered in early life or genetic factors conveying immunity (Douek, et al., 1999).

The protective mechanisms induced by infection that strengthen the immune system are unknown but they are thought to be related to the production of regulatory T-cells (responsible for prompting the immune system to fight infection). The complex interactions between the immune system components that balance this response play a role in the development of both asthma and Type 1 diabetes (Hsia, et al., 2015). This is because the immune response becomes altered and begins to attack both the infection and the body's own insulin-producing cells, or responds adversely to a trigger such as house dust in the case of asthma. Patients with both conditions exhibit lower levels of these components that bring equilibrium to the immune system so that it works effectively, upsetting this unique balance (Marianna, et al., 2006). For this reason, it is therefore likely that both Type 1 diabetes and asthma overlap in patient populations (Hsia, et al., 2015).

Yung-Tshung, et al. (2015) found a significantly higher incidence (the number of new cases) of asthma in people with Type 1 diabetes than in the general population. The risk of developing asthma was found to be highest in young people under eight years of age, and interestingly patients who had been periodically hospitalised for their diabetes more than twice per year were more likely to become asthmatic. Those patients with diabetes with less than two visits per year were found not to be at increased risk. This finding implies that the immune system is adversely affected by the severe metabolic upset that is ketoacidosis, requiring the individual with Type 1 diabetes to be hospitalised to reverse the altered pH balance associated with dangerously prolonged hyperglycaemia during infection or deliberate and frequent insulin omission

The increasing number of individuals with Type 1 diabetes who also develop asthma may be explained by a lesser exposure to immune-system strengthening factors at a younger age. As has been suggested, poor glycaemic control may be a contributory factor by increasing susceptibility to further auto-immune attack by impairing the already dysfunctional immune system. It is known that poor glycaemic control causes chronic inflammation, upsetting the balance between regulatory T-cell responses. We have also seen the association between periodic hospitalisation for diabetes (meaning ketoacidosis and hyperglycaemia) and an increase in subsequent diagnoses of asthma (Yung-Tshung, et al., 2015). Both Type 1 diabetes and asthma share the same risk factors and a low body weight in childhood has also been suggested as a reason why a child with Type 1 diabetes may go on to develop asthma (Black, et al., 2011).

It is also the case that young persons with both conditions tend to have higher average HbA1c levels than those with Type 1 diabetes alone (Black, et al., 2011). Poorer pulmonary function among people with diabetes has also been noted when compared with non-diabetic individuals (Walter, et al., 2003). Hsia, et al. (2015) have stated that the existence of auto-immune dominated disease does not reduce the incidence of asthma, indicating a common environmental factor behind the disease processes.

The hygiene hypothesis proposes that infections in early childhood may reduce the risk of allergic diseases by strengthening the immune system's defence (Alves, et al., 2007) and this may provide an explanation for the development of auto-immune conditions.

Arthritis

Osteoarthritis is a very common condition in the elderly due to wear and tear of the bones and joints, most commonly the weight-bearing knees and hips, and in younger people this develops in bone following trauma, e.g., a broken wrist. Extra bone then forms to compensate for this degeneration which narrows the spaces between the joints, and cysts also form under the bone surface. The disease is treated with anti-inflammatory medication and physiotherapy to manage the stiffness (Prime, 1987).

Because having diabetes affects bone metabolism, changes to the structure of the skeleton are more common than in the non-diabetic population. Diabetes may affect the musculo-skeletal system in a number of ways, influenced by the breakdown of proteins into glucose (glycosylation), damage caused by abnormal blood glucose levels to nerves and blood vessels, and the accumulation of strengthening collagen which changes the structure of connective tissues (Kim, et al., 2001). This complication is most frequently seen in people who have had Type 1 diabetes for a long duration, although they may also be seen in those with Type 2 in association with increased stress on the joints where there is also obesity.

The joints of the hands are affected in a number of ways, but in terms of auto-immune arthritic changes associated with diabetes, stiffening and limited mobility of the small joints due to over-production of collagen and joint degeneration (known as cheiroarthopathy) is found in 50 percent of people with Type 1 diabetes (Arkkila, et al., 1994) and Type 2 patients (Arkkila, et al., 1997). The condition is not painful but is associated with an increased risk of developing proliferative retinopathy and neuropathy in patients with Type 1 or Type 2 diabetes. In the case of Type 2, cheiroarthopathy is also associated with macrovascular (large blood vessel) disease and poor glycaemic control. Stiffening of the joints in the fingers is exclusively seen in diabetes and can occur after the diagnosis of Type 1 in young persons (Clarke, et al., 1990) as well as in those with a long duration of the disease. Treatment in severe cases consists of corticosteroid injections and surgery to reduce the overgrowth of collagen in these joints (Aljanlan, et al., 1999).

A form of arthritis known as calcific periarthritis is also known to affect the shoulder joints of people with and without diabetes, where there are deposits of calcium in the soft tissues around the joint; a condition often occurring in association with metabolic disturbances such as diabetes (Lehmer and Ragsdale, 2012).

The most frequent arthritic changes to occur in the feet of people with diabetes are the conditions diabetic osteoarthropathy and Charcot neuropathic arthropathy. A link has been made between Type 2 diabetes, obesity and osteoarthritis in the weight-bearing bones of the feet (Kim, et al., 2001). Charcot joints (neuropathic arthropathy) describes the degeneration of the joints of the foot, but the condition has also been seen in the knees, wrists, elbows, shoulders, and intervertebral joints (Sinha, et al., 1972). These arthritic changes affect the individual's gait and change the shape of the foot causing mobility and footwear problems as the following comment from an individual who developed Charcot joints shows:

I woke one morning to find my left foot had swollen to twice the normal size. My doctor and diabetes consultant had no advice other than to rest it, which was impossible as I was working and a busy parent. After a year and a half, the swelling finally went down and I was left with arthritic claw toes and a huge pressure point under the toes on the sole of my foot. It's painful to walk and the changes are permanent. I find this very depressing and very difficult to accept.

Psoriasis

Psoriasis is an auto-immune condition that affects the skin and joints, causing red, flaky, crusty patches covered with silvery scales appearing on the elbows, knees, scalp and lower back, and joint degeneration. These skin patches can become itchy and sore. Whilst Type 2 diabetes is not an auto-immune condition, it is now recognised that psoriasis is associated with an increase in the production of insulin to reduce blood glucose levels and the subsequent development of this form of diabetes (Fitzgerald, et al., 2014). More recently there has been a better understanding of how psoriasis may develop when there is comorbid disease such as Type 2 diabetes. Several studies have shown that obesity (defined as a body mass index of 30>) increases the risk of developing moderate to severe psoriasis (Bremmer, et al., 2010; Sterry, et al., 2007). Additionally, psoriasis has been linked to metabolic syndrome: a group of physical states and cardiovascular risk factors including abdominal obesity; impaired glucose regulation; high levels of triglyceride blood fats; reduced high-density lipid blood fats; and high blood pressure (Jensen, et al., 2013; Tam, et al., 2008; Cohen, et al., 2007; Wakkes, et al., 2007; Eckel, et al., 2005).

Patients with Type 1 diabetes and Type 2 diabetes who also have psoriasis are at increased risk of experiencing cardiovascular events at earlier onset (Mehta, et al., 2010; Tobin, et al., 2010; Neimann, et al., 2006). For those with pre-diabetes, growing evidence shows that psoriasis is more likely to develop when insulin resistance is present (Brauchli, et al., 2008; Boencke, et al., 2007). Insulin resistance is defined as the phenomenon where there is reduced glucose absorption by cells stimulated by insulin (Boencke, el al., 2011). Blood glucose levels then rise, stimulating the pancreatic beta-cells to produce more insulin in an effort to reverse this state although there are already abnormally high insulin levels present which cannot be utilised. The beta cells effectively become over-worked and eventually fail, at which point Type 2 diabetes will develop. This sequence of events highlights the state of insulin resistance as a pre-emptive stage in the development of Type 2 diabetes.

The National Psoriasis Foundation now recommend that fasting blood glucose levels in patients with psoriasis be evaluated at least every five years or every two years if risk factors are present, with a target level of <5.6 mmol/L or 100mg/dl (Bremmer, et al., 2010; Kimball, et al., 2008). However, for a patient with psoriasis and pre-diabetes, this may be very difficult to achieve as this is classed as normoglycaemia (a normal level of blood glucose within acceptable limits of 4.0–7.0 mmol/L), achievable only with very good insulin or blood-glucose lowering medication and diligent diabetes self-management. The consequences of insulin resistance in people with psoriasis are now better understood. It is known that the insulin receptors in cells are signalled by a protein that normally acts to induce glucose uptake in fat cells and promote the widening of blood vessels (vasodilation) in the endothelial cells lining the intestinal tract cells (Hogan, 2011). With decreased sensitivity to insulin, levels of this signalling protein are also reduced, and many other alterations in body chemistry that are specific to people with psoriasis occur in association with insulin resistance.

Because of decreased sensitivity to insulin in cases of psoriasis, vaso-constriction of the arteries (narrowing) occurs leading to earlier artery disease (Balchi, et al., 2010; Karadag, et al., 2010). In obese patients with psoriasis and insulin resistance, adipose (fat) tissue macrophages (cells that remove bacteria and foreign bodies from blood and tissues) can also significantly undermine glucose metabolism to contribute to the development of Type 2 diabetes.

Substances called resistin, adiponectin, adipokines and leptin are also present in abnormal quantities in association with obesity. Resistin is a substance released by the fat cells that, as the name suggests, 'resists' the action of insulin on the cells, preventing the lowering of blood glucose. Levels of resistin are raised in psoriasis and diminished with phototherapy, a treatment commonly used to improve the condition (Boehncke, et al., 2012), High levels of resistin increase the risk of insulin resistance and Type 2 diabetes as with obesity there is more fat tissue.

Leptin is a hormone made by fat cells that is involved in the regulation of body fat. Leptin deficiency is a pathological cause of obesity, although when the obesity is due to excess food consumption and a sedentary lifestyle, leptin levels are high (hyperleptinaemia) and this is a risk factor for type 2 diabetes (Klok, et al., 2007). Patients with psoriasis have been found to have higher leptin levels when compared to those without the condition (Chen, et al., 2008; Johnston, et al., 2008; Wang, et al., 2008).

Adiponectin is a hormone produced by the fat cells that causes sensitivity of tissues to insulin. It has both anti-inflammatory and anti-atherogenic effects [reducing fatty deposits in the arteries] (Takahashi, et al., 2008). However, patients with both type 2 diabetes and psoriasis have lower levels of adiponectin (Fitzgerald, et al., 2014). Although low levels of adiponectin have been found in patients with Type 2 diabetes and psoriasis, no connection has been made regarding the causality or severity of either chronic health condition (Shibata, et al., 2009; Takahashi, et al., 2008). Adipokines are produced by fat cells and are known to cause Type 2 diabetes, high blood pressure and narrowing of the arteries. While there is clearly a link between the adipokines produced by an excess of fat tissue and insulin resistance in Type 2, the association between psoriasis and diabetes independent of obesity is not explained by the presence of adipokines.

It is now believed that the inflammatory molecules associated with psoriasis may not only antagonise the effects of insulin, but also adversely contribute to the development of insulin resistance (Fitzgerald, et al., 2014). Inflammatory processes also contribute to the development of atherosclerotic plaque in the arteries and ongoing inflammation (Hogan, et al., 2011). Atherosclerosis (narrowing) due to plaque formation is also a chronic complication of diabetes, eventually leading to coronary heart disease. A further inflammatory antagonist is interleukin-6 which is also associated with glucose intolerance (Eder, et al., 2009), this being raised when there is coexisting obesity and psoriasis and increasing further as psoriasis worsens (Coimbra, et al., 2010) therefore causing a cyclically damaging effect. Because of the action of interleukin-6 and changes to beta (insulin-producing) cell function, the risk of developing Type 2 diabetes is increased. Blood-glucose lowering medications to treat Type 2 diabetes (Exenatide and Liraglutide) have been found to reduce itching, inflammation and insulin resistance in cases of psoriasis. This is possibly because excess glucose is a toxin in the body, causing irritation and itching.

Because psoriasis can be a seen by others and has the potential to cause painful joints unsurprisingly it is a very distressing auto-immune condition resulting in psychological consequences. It is known that excessive worry makes psoriasis worse (Fortune, et al., 2003). Studies have shown that 37–88 percent of patients feel their psoriasis is caused or worsened by stress (Al'Abadie, et al., 1994; Fortune, et al., 1998; Gupta, et al., 1989). Verhoeven et al. (2009a) confirmed that the stressful effects of daily living mediate increased itching and the worsening of psoriasis, and in a further study showed that very worried patients had an increased susceptibility to the effects of stress (Verhoeven et al., 2009b). The hormonal response to stress involves an increase in histamine levels and inflammatory substances by the immune system, triggering 'sickness behaviour' and depressive symptoms.

Sickness behaviour has been defined as a co-ordinated set of behaviour changes that develop in all cases of illness and include low motivation to eat, listlessness, fatigue, malaise, a reduced interest in social activity, a change in sleep patterns, an inability to experience pleasure, an exag-gerated response to pain and a lack of concentration (Dantzer, 2004; 2001). These behavioural changes are the same as those experienced by an individual with depression although, if triggered by illness, there is a reason for the behavioural change. Conversely, a diagnosis of clinical depression is based on there being no discernible reason for symptoms, such as illness or bereavement.

The prevalence of depression in people with psoriasis is thought to be as high as 30 percent (Weiss, et al., 2002). Other studies have shown the percentage as 38 percent in a sample of 140 patients (Fortune, et al., 2000), and Gupta, et al. (1993) found that 5.5 percent of patients with psoriasis had suicidal thoughts with 9.5 percent expressing their wish to die. A UK study of 146,042 psoriasis patients showed an increased number of diagnoses of depression, anxiety and suicidality when compared to individuals without the condition (Kurd, et al., 2010). It has been estimated that there are over 10,400 diagnoses of depression, 7,100 diagnoses of anxiety, and 350 diagnoses of suicidality attributable to psoriasis each year (Kurd, et al., 2010).

A recent study by Mizra, et al. (2012) stated that the patient's health beliefs about their psoriasis were responsible for the psychological distress they experienced, identifying three cognitive pathways a patient may associate with: vulnerability to harm, defectiveness, and social isolation-predicted anxiety and depression. Although there is strong evidence supporting the presence of depression and anxiety in patients with psoriasis, much of the guidance regarding diagnosis and management fails to include routine screening for anxiety and depression meaning that patients may not receive the support they require.

In terms of treatment options for patients with psoriasis and depressive symptoms, TNF-a medication antagonists are used to supress the immune system response that causes inflammation of the skin. The levels of this substance are also raised during a period of depression (Himmerich, et al., 2008) and have been linked to fatigue and sleepiness, potentially explaining the association between depression and fatigue (Illman, et al., 2005; Patarca, et al., 1994). TNF-a antagonists have been shown to be both safe and beneficial in improving physical and psychological symptoms of psoriasis (Revicki, et al., 2008; Shikar, et al., 2007; Gordon, et al., 2006). There is also evidence that depression in patients with psoriasis may be reversed with this treatment (Kimball, et al., 2012; Himmerbach, et al., 2008; Tyring, et al., 2006).

Psoriasis patients treated with anti-depressant and corticosteroid medication also showed improvement in their physical and psychological symptoms compared with corticosteroid use alone (Alpsoy, et al., 1998). However, evidence has shown that the anti-depressant Fluoxetine, suggested by Lustman, et al. (2006) as being very suitable for the treatment of depression in people with diabetes, has been shown in some studies to exacerbate symptoms of psoriasis (Tan, et al, 2010; Tamer, et al, 2009; Hemlock, et al, 1992). This is also the case with Bupropion (Cox, et al, 2002) and lithium (Basayari, et al, 2010).

There have been very few psychological interventions directed at the effect of stress on psoriasis, or the adverse results of stress on the immune system. Psychological interventions can be divided into those addressing cognitive and behavioural processes (cognitive behaviour therapy) and those targeting a reduction in stress (arousal reduction). One available analysis of eight psychological interventions targeting patients with skin conditions (Lavda, et al., 2012) showed that these studies tended to be small and were not rigorously designed. It was also the case that psychological interventions with differing aims were included, meaning the effects could not be compared with one another. The experience of one person with Type 2 diabetes and psoriasis who had received cognitive behavioural therapy to target stress is as follows:

> I saw a clinical psychologist when my psoriasis was so bad I was taken into hospital and he told me [amongst other observations pertaining to using illness to withdraw from society] that some people regard long-term illness as a sort of place they can retreat into to avoid the world. I hadn't realised that I was doing this and it was true: I stopped going out of the house because people would stare at the peeling scabby patches on my face that I couldn't cover up. I stopped meeting with friends and gave up my job because I thought they wouldn't understand and because my joints hurt so I couldn't move about easily. With strong psoriasis medication and CBT my symptoms improved enough for me to leave hospital after ten weeks.

Chronic complications of diabetes

The most common cause of health problems among individuals with diabetes that are not directly related to auto-immune dysfunction are the numerous chronic complications associated with the condition. An elevated and prolonged blood glucose level prior to the diagnosis of either Type 1 or Type 2 diabetes, or due to poor control of the condition once it is recognised, is the trigger for these secondary severe complications in the long-term such as kidney and eye disease, nerve damage, and cerebrovascular and heart disease. In general, every percentage point drop in HbA1c blood test result (e.g., from 8.0 percent to 7.0 percent) can reduce the risk of microvascular complications (eye, kidney, and nerve diseases) by 40 percent (Stratton, et al., 2000; Diabetes Control and Complications Trial Research Group, 1993). Among people with diabetes, annual eye and foot examination can reduce vision loss and lower-extremity amputations. Detecting and treating diabetic eye disease with laser therapy can reduce the development of severe vision loss by an estimated 50–60 percent (Kung, et al., 2008). Comprehensive foot care programmes can reduce amputation rates by 45–85 percent (Litzelman, et al., 1993; Bild, et al., 1989).

The prevalence of chronic complications is high as the recommended HbA1c of less than 7.0 percent is often difficult to achieve for most people with diabetes. A study of prevalence in Type 2 diabetes by Litwak, et al. (2013) showed that of 66,726 people, 27.2 per cent had macrovascular complications and 53.5 per cent had microvascular complications. Sun, et al. (2011) reported that of 351 people with Type 1 diabetes with an average 50-year duration; 57.4 percent had proliferative retinopathy; 13.1 percent had nephropathy; 60.6 percent had neuropathy; and 48.5 percent had cardiovascular disease. Despite the prevalence of complications among people with either Type 1 or Type 2 diabetes, very little research has been published concerning the psychological effect on the individual. The vast majority of papers on the subject focus on good diabetes self-management in order to prevent the development of complications, leading the author to believe that the subject of having complications amounts to victim blaming the individual as complications develop anyway over time.

It has long been known that prolonged and untreated hyperglycaemia triggers the development of diabetic complications. These eventually occur due to the body's reaction to large amounts of glucose in the cells which is toxic and cannot be effectively dealt with. A potential cause of chronic diabetic complications concerns the way glucose is metabolised by the body. As energy is produced, carbon dioxide and water are released. However, in the presence of large amounts of glucose which impairs the function of cells, it is metabolised into sorbitol (Barnett and Grice, 2011). This substance accumulates in the body's tissues and causes damage as the fluid balance inside and outside the cells is equalised and because the large sorbitol molecules cannot pass through the cell membrane, becoming trapped. The result is damage and death of body cells. (Sorbitol used as an artificial sweetener does not have this effect in the body). This disruption to metabolic processes and the continual presence of excessive glucose appear to be a causative factor in the development of chronic complications. It is also understood that genetic factors may lead to complications for individuals with diabetes, even in those people who maintain their blood glucose levels within normal limits (Barnett and Grice, 2011).

Despite the fact that chronic complications are known to occur more often in those with long-duration diabetes due to altered metabolic control (Sun, et al., 2011) and the fact that complications can still develop in people with well-controlled diabetes, information about how people accept and cope with their further disability is sparse. The intervention of health professionals may have a bearing on this issue as once complications are present they may be improved with better glycaemic control but they cannot be completely reversed. However, the patient's perspective warrants research and indicates a need for psychological assistance as demonstrated by the following comments from individuals with diabetes and complications:

I have Type 2 diabetes and I've also had two heart attacks. I've been told by nurses and doctors that it's my own fault because of my often high blood sugars. Because there is nothing anyone can do now I'm not at the prevention stage for complications I just think I've been left on the scrap heap.

My diabetes is Type 1 and I've had it since I was a baby. After 40 years I've got some retinopathy and nerve damage. One diabetes consultant told me I had done very well to only have mild complications after such a long time, but other hospital staff seem to blame me when I tell them, for example, when I had my recent eye check at the hospital. I have learned to live with the pains in my feet and loss of some sight because it happened gradually and I just got used to it.

I woke up one morning and I was blind. I was devastated and it took me a long time to come to terms with the fact there was nothing I could do about it (although I still haven't really) – diabetes has robbed me of my sight. I was given practical help – white stick, guide dog, taught braille etc., but no help with my emotions. I am angry that this has happened to me, hate myself for not taking better [diabetes] care when I had the chance, and bitter that I lost a job I loved because I couldn't manage. I was told it would take time to adjust, but that was a couple of years ago and I seem stuck at being angry and bitter so my personality's changed.

I've got autonomic nerve damage because I had repeated ketoacidosis as a child. It's affected my digestive system and I now have delayed stomach emptying. Trying to give myself the right insulin to suit my rate of digestion is a hit and miss affair with lots of hypos and hypers. I know there's nothing I can do and it makes me very depressed. I've contemplated suicide several times but I feel that would be selfish and can't bring myself to go through with it. I just have to live with this nightmare that even my diabetes consultant doesn't get because I don't have the same symptoms as other people.

Peripheral neuropathy and depression

Peripheral neuropathy is a chronic complication of diabetes which occurs in two forms: diffuse neuropathy, commonly appearing as disorders of sensation in the extremities of the body; and distal polyneuropathy, affecting many nerves of the hands and feet. A Victorian physician, Frederick Pavy (Pavy, 1885), gave a concise description of the symptoms of peripheral neuropathy in the lower extremities that he had observed in his patients with Type 2 diabetes and high blood glucose levels (remembering that there was no effective treatment for either Type 1 or Type 2 diabetes at that time):

> [Patients present with] Heavy legs, numb feet, lightening pain and deep-seated pain in the feet, extreme sensitivity to touch, muscle tenderness, and impairment of knee tendon reflexes.

It is recognised that those suffering neuropathic pain due to nerve damage in diabetes should receive some degree of psychological support as depression is common in this group (Vileikyte, et al., 2005). A study by de Groot, et al. (2001) supports the relationship between the chronic pain of diabetic peripheral neuropathy and depression, although other debilitating aspects of diabetic neuropathy which may induce depressive symptoms such as unsteadiness on the feet and mobility limitations have not been widely studied. Depression is also and unsurprisingly more likely to occur in those with a long-duration of diabetes and other chronic complications associated with or as a result of the condition.

Pain due to diabetic neuropathy is difficult to measure because it is a subjective occurrence. Many factors may affect the degree of pain experienced, including the individual's tolerance to pain, the severity of neuropathy, the presence of other illness and the personal coping mechanisms employed. It is also the case that the presence of interleukin-6 increases the inflammatory response by the immune system in severe illness. It is thought that this response is associated with the development of depressive symptoms previously described as 'sickness behaviour' whereby both pain and depression manifest (Danzer, 2001). Vileikyte, et al.

(2005) have suggested that the unpredictability of peripheral neuropathy pain and its varying duration is a major factor linked to depression associated with this condition.

Mood change associated with hyperglycaemia

As glucose is toxic to the body in excess it is not surprising that the brain struggles to function when glucose levels are either too high or too low, affecting mood by causing irritability, reducing wellbeing and cognitive dysfunction in people who have Type 1 or Type 2 diabetes. A study by Sommerfield, et al. (2004) using a questionnaire and by setting various tasks showed that short-term hyperglycaemia in people with Type 2 diabetes slows down the speed of decision-making, impairs working memory and some aspects of attention and had a profound effect on mood status. This is also true of people with acute hyperglycaemia in Type 1 diabetes. Glucose is the primary energy source for the brain which requires an uninterrupted and steady supply to avoid disruption to cerebral function. When blood glucose is acutely high or low, the brain suffers with shock. For those with Type 2 diabetes and intermittent or chronic hyperglycaemia, an additional multiple risk of vascular disease (such as stroke) is present due to metabolic syndrome.

Two studies examining the effects of hyperglycaemia on the brain have reported confusion over words and a reduced intelligence (Davis, et al., 1996; Holmes, et al, 1983). These studies were respectively of children with Type 1 diabetes and adults with either Type 1 or Type 2 diabetes. Other research has shown no measurable effect of hyperglycaemia on cognitive function in those with Type 1 diabetes (Draelos, et al., 1995; Gschwend, et al., 1995; Hoffman, et al., 1989) or mood (Weinger, et al., 1995). A further study of people without diabetes showed that a short-term high blood glucose reading of 17.8 mmol/L (320 dl/L) using an insulin clamp to prevent it from reducing blood glucose resulted in increased sensory nerve conduction and reduced motor nerve function (Sindrup, et al., 1988). This demonstrates that high blood glucose levels have an effect on brain function in both diabetic and non-diabetic individuals. The following comments give the individual's perspective:

> I have very difficult to control Type 1 diabetes meaning my blood sugar is either too high or too low most of the time and rarely in the middle where it should be. I sometimes find that I have hyperglycaemia for days and for no particular reason and it makes me very short-tempered with everything and everyone. I am also slow to reply if I'm asked something and I always have a terrible headache, so doing even the simplest things becomes difficult and I often do them wrongly. If I'm writing on the computer I find my words come out muddled and I make a lot of spelling mistakes.

> It's like a vicious circle – I find my blood is high and that makes me lazy and tired so I don't want to do anything. I've got Type 2 so I only have my tablets to bring the sugar down, but I've been told to stick to my dose and not to take extra ones. They told me to do exercise if my thoughts are slow and everything's an effort, or if I find that my blood sugar is too high (I got myself a testing meter because I wasn't given one). They also said I just need to cut down on what I eat to stop me feeling depressed, but I think I eat because I'm depressed, which doesn't help my diabetes.

> I'm like Jekyll and Hyde with my diabetes [Type 1]. When I'm hypo or hyperglycaemic I'm so nasty to the people I love and say really horrible things, flying into rages, stomping around, throwing things, and making a big deal about silly little things. Like one time the tea-towel wasn't folded straight so that became a priority when my husband was worried, telling me to go and test to see if I was high or low and do something about it. Fortunately, he knows that isn't really me and says I can't help it, but I absolutely hate myself afterwards and keep on apologising for being so horrible.

CHAPTER 6

DIABETES DEBATE

Type 2 diabetes is recognised as a chronic health condition which is thought to occur in 90 percent of cases because the individual has a high fat, high carbohydrate diet accompanied by little or no exercise. On an individual basis there is reported stigma that the condition is regarded by society as 'self-induced'. Some people with Type 2 have stated that they feel they are blamed by health professionals and misunderstood by those with Type 1 diabetes whose condition is due to autoimmune disease and not lifestyle choice. The following comments from people with Type 2 diabetes demonstrate this:

> I was once at a diabetes clinic and a woman actually started shouting at me, saying there was nothing she could do about her Type 1 diabetes and that I was lucky because all I had to do was lose weight to get rid of my Type 2.

> Several times I've been told by nurses, doctors and dieticians that it is all in my own hands and that I've made myself like this because I've got no self-control or motivation to exercise, and that I obviously don't care about my body and what I eat.

This raises the question of whether it is possible to change eating and exercise behaviour in order to reverse the life-threatening consequences of Type 2 diabetes. Do people actually understand what the condition involves, despite receiving diabetes health education? The enormity of secondary diabetes complications and the need for continual vigilant self-care is a daunting prospect for the newly diagnosed and often a depressing burden for those with long-duration diabetes. Although the author has had very difficult to control Type 1 diabetes for almost 40 years I admit that as a young person I had a complete lack of understanding and total denial of my condition for around fifteen years. Whilst complications do actually catch up eventually if there are dangerous and continual fluctuations in blood glucose levels, I exacerbated sight impairment and nerve damage by just not caring about diabetes as a child. There has never been a better time to be diagnosed with diabetes in terms of the medical profession's current knowledge and understanding of this condition and the help that is now available. The subject of why individuals with diabetes do and do not engage in trying to manage their condition in the best way possible according to their personal circumstance is therefore of great interest to me.

Type 2 diabetes: a growing epidemic

In recent years the number of people developing Type 2 diabetes in the United Kingdom has soared by 65 percent so that 3.5 million are now living with the condition. The symptoms of both Type 1 and Type 2 are similar because they are both due to high levels of glucose in the body: excessive urination and excessive thirst, which is the body's attempt to flush out the glucose it cannot use as fuel as a waste product. Symptoms appear such as tiredness, frequent urination, blurred vision, slow healing of wounds, and numbness in the feet and legs. However, Type 2 diabetes may develop very gradually, as we have seen, over as long as 12 years because the symptoms are milder than in Type 1 diabetes (World Health Organisation 2011; Diabetes UK, 2008).

As the onset of the disease is slow, these symptoms may go unrecognised or may be tolerated by the individual for many years before consulting a doctor. It is also the case that Type 2 diabetes, or being at high risk of developing the condition, may only be picked up during a routine blood test or visit to the doctor. However, complications of diabetes due to high and continual blood glucose levels, such as eye, heart or kidney disease may have already begun before diagnosis of the primary condition.

The current Type 2 diabetes epidemic is fuelled by physical inactivity and obesity as these are the primary risk factors for developing metabolic syndrome, insulin resistance/pre-diabetes, and eventually Type 2 diabetes. The problem is now so great that health professionals in the UK cannot keep up with the number of new diagnoses. For those who have received Type 2 diabetes information, education and support this assumes that the individual is then equipped to manage their condition as well as they can. The following comments are from people with Type 2 diabetes who have recently undergone the associated DESMOND training (Diabetes Education and Self-Management for Ongoing and Newly Diagnosed). Clearly they do not represent the individuals who have read around the subject and have fully embraced the challenge of a Type 2 diabetes diagnosis. However, they suggest that for a section of the Type 2 population, there is insufficient information about the condition available via the training course in terms of difficulties with acceptance and adjustment to having this condition, poor understanding of what this involves; and a lack of knowledge and motivation to manage it as well as possible:

> I was just told that foods are like a sort of traffic light system: vegetables are good; pasta, potatoes and bread in moderation; cakes and sweets never. There was no explanation of how glucose is used by the body and that when I have a hypo, I need to boost my blood glucose with something sweet. I only know this because my friend's child is a Type 1 diabetic.

> I was told to attend this diabetes course by my GP. I was still in shock that I even had diabetes, and they didn't seem to understand that. It was all about what I had to give up if I wanted to stay alive and, after about half an hour, I just walked out.

> I know I should be good but sometimes I eat something naughty because life's too short to deny yourself all the time. I don't really understand why it matters apart from that I might get heart disease one day. Well, I might get that anyway...

Conversely individuals who had recently undergone the DAFNE (Dosage Adjustment For Normal Eating) training for people diagnosed with Type 1 diabetes appeared to have a better understanding of effective diabetes self-management and the reasons for it:

> It's great to know I can give myself an amount of insulin for a specific food and then eat it, not like when I just had two injections a day and had to watch what I ate. Now I can be normal again!

> It makes so much sense – your body produces insulin to cover the food you eat. This way, after calculating the carbohydrate value, you get the correct amount of insulin rather than a standard dosage. This means I can be more flexible with my diet and I also have much better glucose control.

> I'm very keen to minimise any complications if I can and I don't want to take my eye off the ball. It's important to look after yourself. I've got a friend with Type 2 who eats what she likes and says she doesn't care if she dies a bit earlier because of it, as long as she's enjoyed her life. But I can't understand why someone with diabetes wouldn't want to do that.

Providing information to patients does not necessarily translate directly into increased knowledge. What the individual understands about a certain topic comes from many sources. In the case of diabetes, the individual may have friends and family with the condition from whom they develop a perception of what it is like to live with the disease.

Diabetes is also frequently portrayed for dramatic effect in films, television soap operas and books with the aim of educating viewers and readers about the condition via a character. However, these portrayals are often over-dramatised and do not reflect the reality of living with diabetes. Therefore, the individual's idea of what having diabetes might entail, and how to cope with it, is shaped by a number of sources and not just a leaflet from the doctor or diabetes clinic. Whilst there is a lot to take in with a diagnosis of diabetes, comments from the following individuals with Type 2 diabetes imply that it might not be taken as seriously as having Type 1:

> Type 2 diabetes – is that my sugar levels?

> I take my diabetes tablets and then I eat what I like. But sometimes, when I eat doughnuts, I feel unwell and have to have a lie down and have a sleep.'

> I have diabetes, but it's only Type 2 so it's not very serious.

> I have carbohydrate-intolerant diabetes.

Management of Type 2 diabetes

Type 2 diabetes usually occurs in individuals who are over the age of 40 (Diabetes UK, 2012) although it is now becoming worryingly more common in children and young adults. Type 2 diabetes develops because of a group of adverse physical changes and cardiac risk factors which includes abdominal obesity, impaired glucose regulation, high blood fats, reduced high-density lipids, and hypertension. Insulin resistance means that glucose absorption by cells (stimulated by insulin) is reduced. Although a range of factors contribute to a diagnosis of Type 2 diabetes (such as fatty liver disease and metabolic syndrome), the major risk factor is obesity which counts for 80–85 percent of overall risk and underlies the current worldwide epidemic of the condition (Diabetes UK, 2012). Whilst this is the case, obesity does not cause Type 2 diabetes and it should be noted that the condition also develops in those who are not obese. Conversely, individuals who are obese do not automatically develop Type 2 diabetes.

It is known that both genetic and environmental factors play a part in the risk of developing Type 2, meaning that those with close family members who have the condition are 2–6 times more likely to develop the condition than the general population without this familial predisposition (Vaxilliare and Froguel, 2010). Genetic factors also mean that South Asian individuals are six times more likely to develop Type 2 diabetes (predominantly around age 25); whilst those of Afro-Caribbean origin are three times more likely to develop the condition than Caucasian individuals (Department of Health, 2001).

Current Type 2 diabetes management aims to encompass all aspects of the individual's lifestyle and provides a tailored diabetes care plan specific to the person's glucose problems and other health conditions (National Institute for Health and Care Excellence [NICE], 2014a). This includes dietary advice from a nutritional specialist where HbA1c may be set above the 6.5 percent target. This is because patients managing their Type 2 diabetes with diet alone do not take insulin or blood glucose-lowering medication to reduce high glucose levels when necessary. As we have seen, NICE guidance (2014a) recommends that Type 2 patients receive a diabetes management plan tailored to their specific glucose irregularities. However, given the previous comments from Type 2 diabetes patients concerning their own understanding of the condition, and considering the following comments concerning diabetes self-management, this suggests that diabetes health education may be perceived by some as overwhelming, translating into denial or poor motivation for self-care:

> My daughter has Type 1 diabetes and doesn't really look after it properly. When I developed Type 2 last year I knew it wasn't as bad as hers, so I do the same as she does because I don't really want to know.

> Although I probably should, I don't want to read things about diabetes because it just depresses me. It's probably because some-

where in my brain I think if I don't know I can't worry about it, then it doesn't seem like such a big deal.

I'm not going to let having diabetes [Type 2] ruin my life. I eat and drink what I like, when I like as it's too much hassle to be dieting and worrying about what carbohydrates I'm eating and whether I'm having the right amount of exercise or not. I've never had a hypo, so I must be doing OK.

In the absence of glucose-lowering medication, people with Type 2 diabetes are taught to manage the condition with a carbohydrate-restricted diet and regular exercise. However, the individual may not be aware of certain physical responses to exercise when they have diabetes. Intense exercise can cause the liver to release stored glucose (as glucagon), which actually raises blood glucose levels rather than the common misconception that exercise automatically burns glucose and lowers blood glucose levels. This is because glucose is the sole fuel for muscles. When intense exercise is undertaken, there is a seven to eightfold increase in glucose production in the body and glucose utilisation rises three to fourfold (Marliss and Vranic, 2002). This means there may not be enough insulin present to keep glucose levels within range.

The utilisation of glucose is a complex process dependent on regulating influences such as insulin, plasma glucose and muscle factors. When exercise is undertaken, a rise in glucose availability occurs even when additional insulin is taken as this response cannot be avoided. When the body reaches the stage of exhaustion following intense exercise there is therefore substantial hyperglycaemia because less glucose is used than has been produced. The pancreas in a non-diabetic individual produces more insulin for 40–60 minutes after exercise while blood glucose levels are high but because this natural insulin response is absent in people with diabetes, the result is sustained hyperglycaemia if additional insulin or blood glucose–lowering medication is not taken. Exercise-induced hyperglycaemia is therefore commonly reported by individuals with diabetes (Marliss and Vranic, 2002).

Moderate exercise will reduce blood glucose levels but if they are initially high (>15mmol/L or 270 mg/dl) it is not appropriate to exercise as high glucose levels thicken the blood and this exerts a strain on the heart to pump it around the body. In addition, hypoglycaemia due to too much working insulin may ensue if it is administered and exercise is then undertaken. This is because exercise can increase insulin mobilisation from the site at which it is injected so there is more working at one time, particularly if this is in an exercised region such as the arm or leg (Marliss and Vranic, 2002). This results in falling glucose levels that may reach the hypoglycaemic range (depending on the pre-exercise blood glucose level) because the rise in insulin blocks the effect of glucagon on glucose production by the liver. This also increases glucose utilisation to a higher degree than is necessary for the exercise (Marliss and Vranic, 2002).

Obese patients whose blood glucose is not well-controlled by diet and exercise alone are prescribed the glucose-lowering drug Metformin which is also prescribed for the same purpose to those who are not overweight. Because Metformin has gastrointestinal side effects (diahorrea) it is gradually introduced. The drug should also be used with caution for patients who have decreased kidney function, liver dysfunction and cardiac impairment. Annual monitoring of those with Type 2 diabetes should also involve measurement of blood pressure for individuals without hypertension (high blood pressure) or kidney disease, especially when patients have poor glycaemic control. A cardiovascular function and diabetes complications risk assessment is also carried out, as well as management of blood fats, introducing statins to reduce cholesterol levels if necessary. Anti-thrombotic therapy, such as the introduction of a 75mg daily dose of aspirin to prevent blood clots, may also be initiated.

Despite the established guidelines which outline the ongoing checks a person with diabetes should receive, in January 2016 the UK Government announced that diabetes care was a post-code lottery in this respect, stating that huge variations exist in diabetes education, care and management across the country. Whilst people know they have diabetes (although some are unaware if they have Type 1 or Type 2), they may have little understanding of the potential serious consequences of the condition and that it requires both good self-care and healthcare provision that is ongoing. The following comments from people with Type 2 demonstrate a poor understanding of the basics – what diabetes is; how it affects the body; and how and why it must be managed:

> You take the [blood glucose lowering] tablets and feel OK, but I've been told you're not really.

> I don't know if I've got Type 1 or Type 2. I didn't used to have to, but now I inject twice a day and drink a lot of Lucozade because I'm a manual worker and often feel unwell. That's all I know.

> I don't know if I'm Type 1 or Type 2 but I know I feel sick if I eat cake.

Reversal of Type 2 diabetes with diet and exercise

Whilst dietary modification alone does not have a significant effect on Type 2 diabetes, clinical research shows that lifestyle change in addition to weight loss for obese patients can reverse glucose impairment (Ahmad and Crandall, 2010). Behavioural change as an approach to reversing Type 2 diabetes has been documented for over 10 years (Holford, 2011; Boden, et al., 2005; Harder, et al., 2004; Vernon, et al., 2003; Yipp, et al., 2001). An intensive lifestyle change programme in the United States involving a calorie, carbohydrate and fat restricted diet was successful in preventing Type 2 diabetes in obese individuals thought to be at high risk of developing the condition (Mayer-Davis, et al., 2004).

The author has seen five individuals with Type 2 diabetes reverse their condition with complete lifestyle change (not as part of a research study). This was achieved via dietary modification – the avoidance of refined carbohydrates and eating smaller portions – and by taking moderate (not intense) cardiovascular exercise three times a week. The average weight loss was 28 pounds (2 stones) under medical supervision which achieved HbA1c results within normal range. These individuals adopted this lifestyle change and maintained the status without the use of Metformin or insulin for an average of four years. This behaviour change was not permanent for everyone due to a change in circumstances for two people, but this does demonstrate that lifestyle-related Type 2 diabetes can be reversed (with medical guidance), reducing the risk of life-threatening chronic diabetes complications. The reduction in bodyweight must, however, be maintained because the presence of fat impairs the action of insulin and, if weight is regained, Type 2 diabetes returns.

Previous research studies have shown similar findings to that of these five individuals. Westman, et al. (2008) found that 85 patients with Type 2 diabetes who adopted a low-carbohydrate diet of <20g a day for six months but without any calorie restriction achieved reduced blood glucose levels and improved glycaemic control. Because carbohydrates (starches) are converted to glucose by the body, low carbohydrate diets are also low glycaemic index diets which moderate any rise in blood glucose levels. The study found that by eliminating or strictly reducing carbohydrate intake, this reduced or avoided the need to take glucose-reducing medication in motivated research participants. Other studies have had similar outcomes (Boden, et al., 2005; Vernon, et al., 2003). This evidence supports the idea that lifestyle modification can reverse Type 2 diabetes if the individual is sufficiently motivated by the benefits of improved health.

Adopting a very low calorie diet is not the same as healthy eating and/ or reducing carbohydrate intake as low carbohydrate diets may permit a normal fat intake (meaning they are not low in calories). An obese patient may need to lose weight rapidly so that they can undergo surgery (such as joint replacement) and a very low calorie diet of <800 calories a day may be suggested. These diets should only be undertaken for a period of three months under medical supervision (NICE, 2014c) because vitamin and mineral deficiency can develop. If the individual has Type 2 diabetes and chronic complications – such as those with reduced liver or kidney function, cardiac impairment, disordered eating and other psychological health issues – a restricted diet may not be suitable.

Current recommendations from the National Institute for Care Excellence (NICE, 2014c) state that gastric band surgery for weight loss should be offered to more people with Type 2 diabetes to reduce the 5.5 billion pounds per annum cost of treating diabetes. Whilst dietary restriction and exercise may not be suitable for morbidly obese patients, lifestyle change to achieve weight loss is cheaper for the NHS and is associated with far fewer complication risks and side effects than surgery. In order for obese patients to adopt lifestyle change they require motivation and support from the health professionals providing their care. The underlying issues of why the patient overeats also need to be investigated and addressed, as the following comments show:

> With the help of a dietician and a clinical psychologist I discovered that I ate for comfort because I was unhappy. It was a vicious circle because then I was unhappy because I was fat. Once I'd got to the root cause, I realised I was just eating for the sake of it and not because I was hungry. I know this sounds simple but I've managed to lose 3 stone and now my blood glucose control [with Type 2 diabetes] is normal.

> I've had some things happen in my life that I felt were my fault: I was adopted and in care homes for a lot of my childhood. I never connected this with why I enjoyed my food so much. I paid to see a counsellor for three months and got to the bottom of it all. It clicked into place and made sense. Every time I thought about eating junk food I reminded myself of what we'd discussed. My [Type 2] diabetes is now so much better and my consultant is hoping I can eventually come off Metformin completely.

As we have seen, excess body fat impedes the action of insulin on the cells leading to insulin resistance and raised blood glucose levels. Weight loss means that a certain amount of fat is removed from the body so insulin is able to work normally, improving glycaemic control in obese persons with Type 2 diabetes. As has been suggested in the previous patient comments, this can eliminate the need for glucose-lowering medication. A modified diet and regular cardiovascular exercise has the potential to return the individual to a pre-diabetes state without the potentially dangerous side-effects of bariatric surgery. However, this lifestyle change must be tailored to the individual's specific needs by appropriately trained health professionals offering ongoing assistance and encouragement. As with weight loss surgery, diet and exercise is not a quick fix solution and the lifestyle changes adopted must become permanent, with a high degree of motivation from the individual, in order to succeed and experience health benefits.

Bariatric (weight loss) surgery

Obesity, defined as a Body Mass Index (BMI) of 30 kg/m^2 and above, is a chronic condition that is rapidly increasing in adults and children. The World Health Organisation has categorised obesity as an epidemic (World Health Organisation, 2000). It is a significant risk factor for the development of many health conditions including heart disease, Type 2 diabetes, hypertension (high blood pressure), dyslipidemia (abnormal blood fats, such as high cholesterol), stroke, atheroscleroisis (fatty deposits in the arteries), and some types of cancer (Whitlock, et al., 2009). Obesity is not only a risk factor for serious physical disease; it also leads to psychological disorders, disordered eating and an impaired quality of life for the individual, with complications and mortality increasing with the duration of obesity (Kubik, et al., 2013). The morbidly obese, defined as those with a BMI of above 40 kg/m^2, are now a rapidly emerging sub-group.

The National Institute for Health and Care Excellence (NICE, 2014b) has stated that more than a quarter of UK adults are now classed as obese and a further 42 percent of men and a third of women are overweight; and 1 in 6 NHS beds is currently taken up by a person with Type 1 or Type 2 diabetes and complications (NICE, 2014b). It is thought that 1.4 million morbidly obese people could benefit from bariatric surgery, potentially reversing 40,000 cases of Type 2 and 5,000 cases of heart disease as currently 17 billion pounds is spent by the NHS on obesity-related conditions per year. It is clear that a weight loss of 5–10 percent is beneficial in ameliorating chronic health conditions that are exacerbated by excess body fat (Maggard, et al., 2005). Whilst behavioural change to incorporate a healthy lifestyle and moderate exercise is successful for the mild to moderately overweight, this approach is not advisable for the morbidly obese. Weight loss surgery – where a gastric band is fitted to drastically reduce the size of the stomach – is not an easy option and it is not a quick fix. The individual must make significant changes to their diet and exercise behaviour and lifestyle in order for the surgery to be successful as the following comment demonstrates:

> I stuck to the restricted diet after I'd had the surgery for about a month. Then I started to cheat and had lots of ice cream and full-fat coffees because I was miserable, so I actually put the 10 pounds I'd lost back on plus a bit more. I had to eventually admit what I'd been doing and my doctor threatened I'd have to have the band removed if I wasn't going to use it properly. I felt so guilty and ashamed that it forced me to be good.

Bariatric surgery works by restricting the amount of food that can be eaten and by reducing the amount of nutrients that can be absorbed. There are two basic types of bariatric surgery: restrictive surgeries and malabsorptive/restrictive surgeries. Restrictive surgeries work by physically making the size of the stomach much smaller in order to slow down digestion so the patient feels fuller for longer with less food. Malabsorptive/restrictive surgeries are more invasive for the individual because this method involves physically removing a portion of the digestive tract which restricts the absorption of calories.

The insertion of an adjustable gastric band (also known as lap band surgery) is one example of restrictive surgery. Stomach banding is the process of placing a synthetic band around the upper portion of the stomach to form a small pouch just below the oesophagus to significantly reduce the amount of food that can be eaten, therefore reducing calories.

The size of the pouch can be altered by the surgeon by inflating or deflating the band through a port that is implanted beneath the skin on the abdomen. The band can be removed at any time. Other procedures include laparoscopic sleeve gastrectomy – where a small portion of the stomach is sectioned off so that it takes less food to become full – and biliopancreatic diversion – surgery to reduce the size of the stomach and intestine to limit food intake and absorption.

Reversal of Type 2 diabetes with surgery

The reversal of Type 2 diabetes via bariatric surgery to reverse morbid obesity was first observed more than 10 years ago following bariatric surgery (Keidar, 2011). It has been shown unequivocally that certain procedures, such as the Roux-en-Y gastric bypass (RYGBP) and biliopancreatic diversion (BPD), are more effective treatments for the reversal of Type 2 diabetes than traditional weight loss or medication. These methods have proved particularly successful in returning levels of plasma glucose, insulin and HbA1c to normal levels in 80–100 percent of morbidly obese patients (Keidar, 2011).

Studies have shown that normal blood glucose and insulin levels occur within days after surgery, despite the fact that there has been little time for any significant weight loss (Rubiano, et al., 2010a; 2010b; Schernthaner and Morton, 2008; Crookes, 2006; Rubiano, et al., 2006a; 2006b). This evidence suggests that weight loss alone is not the reason insulin can work more effectively as without weight loss its action is still being impaired by fat. It is possible that the results of these studies are due to a combined smaller food intake, reduced malabsorption of nutrients, and the anatomical change in the gastrointestinal (GI) tract affecting glucose metabolism. It is hoped that a better understanding of these mechanisms may mean new treatments for Type 2 diabetes and obesity in the future.

Interventions aimed at healthy eating, regular exercise and behaviour change with the additional use of weight loss medication have been periodically tried to tackle obesity. However, significant weight loss has rarely been achieved, especially in the morbidly obese (Buchwald, 2005; Tsai and Wadden, 2005). These weight loss intervention programmes have proved largely unsuccessful as they do not incorporate restricted eating, with a failure rate of around 95 percent at one year (Keidar, 2011).

Keidar (2011) conducted a systematic analysis of published studies reporting the successful reversal of Type 2 diabetes, describing the discontinuation of medication to lower blood glucose levels and the achievement of normal blood glucose levels in up to 86.6 percent of patients. Following bariatric surgery there was an average weight loss of 38.5 kilograms, equating to almost 56 percent of excess weight (Buchwald, et al., 2009). A further study of the diabetes status of 240 morbidly obese patients after bariatric surgery by Schauer, et al. (2003) showed that 80 percent became diabetes-free with an average weight loss of 60 percent (97 pounds). A previous study of 330 patients who had undergone weight loss surgery by Pories, et al. (1995) reported similar findings and showed normal fasting blood glucose levels without medication in 89 percent of patients. Patients with a short duration (<5 years) of Type 2 diabetes who had formerly been able to control their blood glucose levels with diet and no glucose-lowering medication or insulin achieved the best weight loss and were therefore more likely to have their condition reversed by bariatric surgery.

There is no doubt physiologically that significant weight loss enables insulin to work more effectively to lower blood glucose levels. Two controlled studies examining glycaemic control in morbidly obese patients following their bariatric surgery have shown the extent of this glycaemic improvement. A Swedish study of 641 patients showed that a 16.1 percent weight loss over 10 years resulted in the risk of going on to develop obesity-related Type 2 diabetes was three times lower than in control subjects, and recovery rates from Type 2 diabetes were three times higher than in those who did not have the surgery (Sjöström, et al., 2004).

A further controlled study compared morbidly obese patients with a <2-year duration of conventionally-managed Type 2 diabetes to those who had received bariatric surgery (Dixon, et al., 2008). Results showed significant reductions in fasting blood glucose, HbA1c and the need for glucose-lowering medication. The most impressive results in a study of Type 2 diabetes reversal following bariatric surgery have come from Marinari, et al (2006) who, in a 10-year follow-up of patients, found that 97 percent of the 268 individuals included in the study had achieved and sustained normal blood glucose levels for this period. These studies show that the reversal of Type 2 diabetes following bariatric surgery is not short-term and that normal blood glucose and HbA1c levels can be achieved with this health outcome.

The long-term physical consequence of bariatric surgery on the morbidly obese population has been shown to be so effective it can be stated that mortality is significantly reduced as a result. Adams, et al. (2007) have shown that deaths attributed to Type 2 diabetes were reduced by 92 percent, proving unequivocally that weight loss surgery is an extremely effective treatment for the condition. As a result of this success rate, bariatric procedures are being adopted as a worldwide treatment option for Type 2 diabetes in cases of morbid obesity and, more frequently, overweight patients

Complications following bariatric surgery
Bariatric surgery is associated with the risk of complications, but these vary according to the type of procedure (Crookes, 2006). Because the simpler restrictive procedures (e.g., gastric banding) are less invasive they rarely affect the function of the bowel. This means that there is a reduced risk of malabsorption of nutrients and subsequent vitamin deficiency unless repeated vomiting occurs. Erosion of the band by the hydrochloric acid in the stomach and digestive enzymes has been noted, with this resulting in abdominal pain and impairment of weight loss (Keidar, 2011). Additionally, over-filling of the band has resulted in the band slipping down the stomach, effectively making the pouch available for food larger with either no weight loss or weight gain being reported (Crookes, et al., 2008; Keidar, et al., 2005).

As would be expected, surgical procedures which deliberately restrict the absorption of nutrients can lead to major dietary deficiencies. Surgery designed to cause malabsorption of nutrients is a serious procedure that can lead to short and long-term complications. Problems may occur within the first month following bariatric surgery such as poor wound healing (a particular difficulty in patients with diabetes), and incision hernias (pushing part of the digestive tract out of its normal position) following bypass and re-joining parts of the small bowel to reduce the absorption of nutrients (Podnos, et al., 2003). Obstruction of the small bowel has been reported in 2.1 percent of patients, as had narrowing of the small bowel in 0.7 percent of surgeries; gastrointestinal bleeding in 0.6 percent of patients; leakage of the contents of the small bowel at the surgery site (1.2 percent); blockage of the pulmonary artery by a blood clot (pulmonary embolus) in 1.0 percent of cases; and the onset of pneumonia in 0.1–0.3 percent of patients following gastric bypass procedures (Keidar, 2011).

The majority of later-onset complications following gastric bypass concern the disruptive effect of surgery on the gastro-intestinal tract. As we have already seen, nutritional deficiencies pose a major problem, especially the potential lack of protein-calories (resulting in swelling of the lower limbs and a feeling of weakness); calcium and iron depletion and vitamin deficiencies. This highlights the need for quality nutrition to be taken in the much-reduced portion sizes with the addition of appropriate vitamin supplementation. In this context, Schweiger, et al. (2010) have stated that nutritional deficiencies can develop as a result of anorexia, poor vitamin and mineral supplementation, prolonged vomiting, stricture formation (the growth of scar tissue causing narrowing), or poor intestinal absorption of nutrients.

Berger, et al. (2004) have also associated weight loss surgery with certain neurological complications due to severe vitamin deficiency when there is continual vomiting, such as beri beri (a lack of vitamin B1) causing either heart and circulatory problems or affecting the nerves and depleting muscle strength (depending on whether the condition is wet or dry beri beri respectively); and a condition known as Wernicke's encephalopathy which is a neurological disorder caused by thiamine (vitamin B1) deficiency. Peripheral neuropathy, common in those with diabetes, is a further potential complication of weight loss surgery, as are spinal cord lesions due to vitamin B12 and folic acid deficiency (also known as vitamin B9). Iron and calcium deficiency due to a reduced absorption area in the duodenum and jejunum (the first and second parts of the small intestine) often occurs in female patients of child-bearing age (Coates, et al., 2004; Skroubis, et al., 2002). Osteopenia (loss of bone density) is a consequence of calcium deficiency following gastric bypass surgery, and vitamin D deficiency (essential for a healthy immune system and bone strength in association with calcium) may go unrecognised as it results in generalised muscle pain and weakness.

Symptoms of heartburn and regurgitation have been reported by patients who have undergone malabsorptive/restrictive surgeries (Keidar, et al., 2010; Crookes, et al., 2006). Due to the nature of the surgery, bowel disturbances are commonly experienced by patients following weight loss procedures, although the body adapts to this change over time. When the surgery is restrictive rather than also malabsorptive, patients frequently complain of constipation as there is a reduced volume of food passing through the digestive tract with less fibre content. The formation of gallstones (cholelithiasis) is also a common complication of rapid weight loss for any reason (Keidar, 2011; Crookes, 2006).

Risks: Type 2 diabetes and bariatric surgery

Bariatric surgery is clearly a serious undertaking, but this is especially true if the individual has Type 2 diabetes, which increases the chance of morbidity (disease) and mortality (death) following this procedure. Microvascular changes in people with diabetes lead to poor blood supply which means that wound healing is slow. This has been suggested as a primary reason for the resulting leakage following bariatric procedures involving open and laparoscopic methods (via a small incision into the abdominal cavity) with associated complications (Fernandez, et al., 2004). However, as we have already seen, the need for a reduced intake of food in order to achieve weight loss and the reversal of Type 2 diabetes outweighs the mortality and morbidity risk associated with the surgery itself. This has been demonstrated by Adams, et al. (2007) who reported a reduction of up to 92 percent in deaths from Type 2 diabetes because of achieving reversal of the condition by gastric bypass.

The National Institute for Health and Care Excellence (NICE, 2014b; 2014c) recently updated its guidance on obesity and advised that obese individuals with recently diagnosed Type 2 diabetes should be assessed for weight loss surgery as it is beneficial to both the patient and to the NHS in terms of the associated cost savings. NICE already recommends that people should be offered weight loss surgery if they have a BMI of over 35. Although there is an initial cost to the NHS of around £6,000 per procedure, in the long-term the cost of treating Type 2 diabetes and its complications would be far greater. Therefore, by putting the emphasis on the surgical treatment of Type 2 diabetes before complications arise from prolonged hyperglycaemia, the greater chance that the individual can lead a healthy, active life. The need to prevent complications is demonstrated by the following comments:

> I paid to have weight loss surgery two years ago. I used to take insulin for [Type 2] diabetes and, almost as soon as I'd had the operation, I didn't have to inject any more, even though I hadn't actually lost much weight. Unfortunately, I had already developed eye [retinopathy] and nerve [neuropathy] complications that have not improved or gone away, despite the fact that my blood sugar is now normal and so is my HbA1c.

> I had a heart attack and a gastric band fitted last year. I've lost weight and my diabetes has actually gone, but the years of being an undiagnosed diabetic have caused damage to my heart and circulation that can't be reversed.

In the United States the number of bariatric procedures performed on patients with Type 2 diabetes was estimated at 225,000 per year (Crookes, 2006) although ten years on, this is now much higher. Keidar (2011) has stated that if the number of weight loss surgeries in the US rose to one million per annum, the estimated 1 in 200 risk of death as a result of undergoing this procedure would mean 5,000 expected deaths from surgical complications. Relating this to patients with either Type 1 or Type 2 diabetes, with a mortality rate of three patients per 1,000, this suggests that 15,000 people would die over a 5-year period. Because gastric bypass surgery to treat obesity and Type 2 diabetes is known to reduce diabetes-related deaths by up to 90 percent (Scopinaro, et al., 2005), Keidar (2011) has suggested that 14,310 Type 2 diabetes-related deaths would be prevented by bariatric surgery over this time period. It is clear that morbidly obese patients with Type 2 diabetes can benefit from surgical intervention, but the mortality risks require discussion with the individual in order for them to make an informed decision about whether to go ahead. This process is shown in the following comment:

> I was advised to have surgery to lose weight and help my diabetes. It sounded like a great idea because I've always struggled with my weight and health. Although they explained the risks to me, it didn't really seem real because I didn't know what I'd be facing – a chance of dying just doesn't seem real when you're sitting in the consultant's office nodding at everything you're being told. I just wanted to lose weight and feel better. I did have problems after the operation and I was very ill with a long stay in hospital. If I'd known this would happen [meaning having had the experience rather than just being told] I think I would still have gone ahead, but I didn't know how hard it would be to go without the pleasure of food as it's part of every occasion in life. I miss that, even though my diabetes has gone because I've lost just over five stone.

A study reviewing the typical amount of weight lost following bariatric surgery showed that the average of 47.5 percent excess loss in patients who had a gastric band fitted and 61.6 percent of total bodyweight was shed by the individuals who underwent gastric bypass surgery (Buchwald, et al., 2004). Weight loss tended to reach a plateau at around two years following surgery, and some weight gain had been reported by the third year (Sarwer, et al., 2012). Perhaps more important than weight loss in terms of medical outcome, bariatric surgery has led to the significant reversal of various weight-related health conditions. We have seen that Type 2 diabetes can successfully be addressed with bariatric surgery, even before there is any great weight loss. It has also been shown that metabolic syndrome can be reversed with weight loss surgery and that an early death from metabolic syndrome (with its associated cardiac risk factors) can be avoided (Dixon, et al., 2008; O'Brien, et al., 2006, Sjöström, et al., 1999). By tackling the growing epidemic of metabolic syndrome and Type 2 diabetes, bariatric surgery offers a cost-effective solution to morbid obesity for the NHS before comorbidities develop in the patient (Picot, et al., 2009).

The psychological impact of bariatric surgery
As we have seen, bariatric surgery is an extremely successful way of treating the current health epidemics of morbid obesity and Type 2 diabetes, reversing the latter condition to delay and stabilise chronic and life-threatening complications of the disease. The surgery is regarded as effective when weight loss and diabetes reversal is achieved, but in the light of this success it must be remembered that the individual has to live a life of forced behavioural change which they may not be fully prepared for, despite psychological counselling, affecting their perception of wellbeing.

Whilst the physical complications of bariatric surgery are well documented, the psychological implications are less so. It is known that morbidly obese individuals experience mood disorders, anxiety and low self-esteem and are five times more likely to have suffered from major depression in the previous five years than average weight individuals (Sarwer, et al., 2012). There are a number of reasons why depression is common among morbidly obese individuals. One major factor is body dissatisfaction (Friedman and Brownell, 1995) and this is especially the case in women, thought to be due to pressure to conform to societal norms (Kubik, et al., 2013). There is also a stigma attached to obesity, causing prejudice and discrimination which causes or worsens depression (Kaminsky and Gadaleta, 2002; Stunkard and Wadden, 1992).

There is evidence that morbid obesity equates to poorer socio-economic status in terms of lower household income, lower educational achievement, and that there is a greater likelihood of being single when comparing this group with average weight peers with a similar intellect (Kubik, et al., 2013). Depressive symptoms are further intensified by yo-yo dieting where weight loss attempts fail, heightening feelings of hopelessness and low self-esteem (Wooley and Garner, 1991). Perhaps contributing to the complex decision to go ahead with bariatric surgery, in addition to the physical reasons, depressive symptoms (due to the factors of body image, low self-esteem and stigma) are reported by 20–30 percent of patients at the time of bariatric surgery, with 50 percent citing a life-long history of depression (Sarwer, et al., 2012).

Psychological health is clearly correlated with further weight gain in obese individuals. Abiles, et al. (2010) have shown that patients undergoing bariatric surgery are more likely to suffer psychological distress compared to obese patients who do not have these procedures. The trigger for such patients to initiate bariatric surgery (rather than it be advised by a physician) is a traumatic or distressing event, such as the death of a loved one (Kalarchian, et al., 2007). It is also the case that individuals seeking surgical or medication-based solutions to obesity are more likely to have experienced psychological distress than those of a similar weight who request dietary advice and behavioural therapy for their obesity (Higgs, et al., 1997). Poor psychological health has also been attributed to individuals with Type 2 diabetes in association with obesity (Anderson, et al., 2001; Dew, 1998, Schleifer, et al., 1989). As we have seen previously, the impact of living with comorbidities such as diabetes-related heart disease, blindness, kidney disease, and/or nerve pain (to name but a few consequences of diabetes complications) takes a massive toll on the individual physically and mentally.

As we have already seen, bariatric surgery is the most effective treatment for weight loss in individuals who are classed are morbidly obese. To be eligible for this type of procedure on the NHS the patient must have failed to lose weight with diet and exercise (non-surgical measures) and have a BMI of > 40 or a BMI of above 35 if there is also an obesity-related comorbidity such as Type 2 diabetes (Kubik, et al., 2013). The goal of putting the patient through expensive and potentially life-threatening surgery is to achieve and maintain a substantial weight loss. Because bariatric surgery enforces extreme dietary change it is expected that the individual will adopt lifestyle change regarding their eating and exercise habits. The selection of suitable candidates for weight loss surgery involves an in-depth assessment of the patient's medical, psychological and social issues.

Significant measures are taken to assess the potential psychological impact of bariatric surgery on the individual. There have been various studies and comprehensive reviews stating that weight loss surgery has resulted in an improvement in depressive symptoms, higher self-esteem, health-related quality of life, and a more positive body image (Van Hout, 2006; Van Hout, et al., 2005; Herpertz, et al., 2003; Bocchieri, et al., 2002). A large study of 4.047 Swedish Obese Subjects (SOS) was conducted by Karlsson, et al. (1998) to assess quality of life and eating behaviour following bariatric surgery. This showed a good adaptation to behaviour change and patients reported a substantial decrease in depression and anxiety in the year following the procedure compared to obese individuals who underwent diet and exercise counselling. This positive outcome was confirmed by a systematic review of 40 studies from 1982–2002 (Herpertz, et al., 2003) showing particular improvement of depression and anxiety, classified as axis 1 psychiatric disorders by the American Psychiatric Association (2013) *Diagnostic Statistical Manual of Mental Disorders* [DSM-IV].

It is clear that these psychological benefits were as a result of the individual's weight loss following bariatric surgery. In addition, any reported post-operative weight regain was associated with an increase in depressive symptoms (Bocchieri, et al., 2002). Because depression and anxiety are so common in morbidly obese patients, several studies have suggested that psychological issues can be attributed to the obesity rather than the individual's personality; improvements in psychological health may be due to the degree of weight loss (Mamplekou, et al., 2005; Guisado, et al., 2002; Karlsson, et al., 1998). Taken altogether, this suggests that psychological conditions in the morbidly obese are attributable to their obesity as opposed to the individual's underlying character. However, the complex relationship of factors involved mean that weight loss is not the central issue.

Dymek, et al. (2001) have stated that psychological health benefits are seen in patients who do not lose any weight following bariatric surgery and before the desired outcome of surgery has occurred. The positive effect of mental health is therefore likely to be due to the adoption of a proactive attitude to tackle obesity despite little or no weight loss: it is therefore the expectation that this will happen as a consequence of surgery. Higgs, et al (1997) have also suggested that having bariatric surgery lifts the burden of the distressing event that triggered the patient to seek a surgical solution to life-threatening obesity.

Despite the stunning success rate of bariatric surgery in reversing obesity-related health conditions and improving the patient's overall physical and mental health status, there are still a minority of patients who do not perceive weight loss surgery as a positive experience. Van Hout (2006) and Bocchieri, et al. (2002) have reported the reduction in long-term health gains or no discernible benefit following weight loss surgery. Kubik, et al (2013) has suggested that patients may have unrealistic expectations of a dramatic change in their life following weight loss surgery, effectively setting the patient up for disappointment and having a negative effect on mental health if these expectations are not met, even with significant weight loss. The following comment demonstrates this point:

> I stupidly thought that my life would be different after I went through the surgery and lost weight: that I'd be more popular, that I'd be invited out to parties and be 'the life and soul'. I thought being thin would change everything. In reality my life hasn't changed at all – it's exactly the same except I'm thinner. I still have the same life with the same problems – my elderly mother, my kids, and a lack of support from people. While I've probably got more confidence now to move to another job or house to make a better life, I think I was expecting too much from the surgery and I'm just as miserable.

Bearing this comment in mind, Kubik, et al. (2013) have stated that patients who have undergone bariatric procedures may realise that they cannot attribute underlying emotional disturbance to their weight; additionally, patients may have difficulty coping with negative life events that they are no longer able to attribute to their obesity.

Studies have shown that the decrease in depressive symptoms following bariatric surgery are not lasting. Sanchez-Zaldıvar, et al. (2009) have reported decreasing levels of depression for up to two years following surgery; whilst Frigg, et al. (2004) suggested that there is a post-operative period of four years during which the patient experiences an improvement in their depression. It is also thought that some improvement in depressive symptoms is seen followed by subsequent decline (Kubik, et al., 2013). This state is associated with weight loss followed by weight gain and the patient reaching a plateau where no further weight is lost (Bocchieri, et al., 2002).

Shai, et al. (2003) have suggested that a key factor in boosting the patient's psychological state following bariatric surgery is the positive reinforcement gained through interaction with health professionals during frequent post-operative appointments. This may explain the correlation between depressive symptoms re-appearing and the reduced need for clinic visits as time goes on. Herpertz, et al. (2003) have reported suicide in patients following weight loss surgery, although it is difficult to attribute the cause directly to the effects of the surgery and it is unclear whether rates of suicide in post-bariatric patients are any higher than in the general population. There is therefore a need for ongoing patient follow-up to assess mental health status, even though physical symptoms, such as raised blood glucose levels, may have been long-reversed.

The individual's self-concept

Self-concept is the individual's self-perception. This is shaped by characteristics such as self-esteem, body image, self-confidence, the individual's perception of attractiveness, and their view of their own assertiveness (Kubik, et al., 2013). It is difficult to study these factors because they are subjective and unique to the individual, but the way these self-concepts shape personality can be observed. Bocchieri, et al. (2002) have stated that, despite the lack of studies in this area, the available literature seems to suggests that bariatric surgery increases self-esteem, self-confidence, and personality because of an improved body image and weight loss satisfaction. A problem with excess skin that does not shrink back in line with weight loss has been a cause of significant distress and body image dissatisfaction, reported in 70 percent of bariatric patients (Kinzl, et al., 2013). Despite the fact that Kubik, et al. (2013) have stated that 90 percent of bariatric patients are pleased with their overall appearance, they report that greater satisfaction with body image was expressed by patients who had lost less weight [meaning less loose skin], and that saggy skin was the reason for dissatisfaction in those who had lost more weight. This is shown in the following comments:

> I wasn't expecting to have so much baggy skin hanging every-where. I was told that my skin had been stretched by the fat and that it wouldn't go back naturally. I've lost lots of weight but my body is still ugly. I'm going to have a second operation [further to bariatric surgery] to remove the skin on the underside of my arms in a few weeks. Then there will be more surgery to have my legs

done and a tummy tuck and bottom lift. I'm wondering when it will ever end. And to top it all I'll have horrible scars everywhere rather than the body I dreamed of.

I wanted to fix the problem when I woke up after the surgery – that the fat and the skin would be gone.

These comments highlight the issue of the patient not being prepared for the after effects of extreme weight loss, despite being told by the surgeon that loose skin was to be expected. It may even be appropriate to show anonymous photographs in order to convey understanding of this issue. Despite the fact that psychological counselling regarding post-operative effects is a very important part of weight loss surgery, the patient must unfortunately learn by experience, leading to the level of dissatisfaction demonstrated by the previous comments. Kubik, et al. (2013) pointed out that plastic surgeons should be part of this counselling team because they carry out body contouring surgery to remove excess skin, emphasising that they must make the patient aware of the limitations of this procedure which may not be in line with the patient's expectations. With this in mind it is difficult to assess whether weight loss surgery actually improves personality disorders. Van Hout, et al. (2006) have reported a reduction in neuroticism, defensiveness and immature identity, and increased discipline in bariatric patients. Conversely, Kubik, et al. (2013) found no difference in post-surgery personality traits, suggesting that such disorders were ingrained behaviours of long-duration, being resistant to change.

Disordered eating is known to be a common behaviour in obese individuals and this is especially the case for binge eating, thought to occur in 5–15 percent of this population who have bariatric surgery (Sarwer, 2012). It is difficult to evaluate the concept of binge eating because it relies on self-reporting by the individual and available studies of the subject, meaning the assessment of whether bariatric surgery can rectify the problem of binge eating remains uncertain. One study has suggested that binge eating behaviour is likely to be reversed following surgery as the emphasis is then placed on dietary restriction (Van Hout, et al., 2006). However, whilst eating a large quantity of high-calorie foods may be a physical impossibility with a very small stomach size, as we saw in a comment at the beginning of this chapter, intake of high-fat ice cream can mean that weight loss is undermined as the individual's psychological mind set still has a desire to 'comfort eat'.

Despite the assessment that bariatric surgery can be effective in reversing binge eating behaviour, the same researchers have also stated that many patients continue to experience disturbing eating disorders after surgery such as exerting tight control over what is eaten for fear of weight gain (Sarwer, et al., 2012). Kubik, et al. (2013) have stated that some patients report a loss of control regarding eating and still feel the desire to overeat, only being deterred by the surgical inability and the prospect of vomiting because the stomach becomes over-full. In a further study examining eating behaviour in patients two years after bariatric surgery, some individuals mentioned the use of vomiting (effectively bulimia) in order to maintain their new weight and shape (de Zwaan, et al., 2010). This insight suggests that vomiting is not always an involuntary response by the stomach following bariatric surgery and that the patient is suffering from a psychologically significant eating disorder.

Weight loss surgery in children

There are now escalating cases of children, traditionally only developing Type 1 diabetes, who are now developing Type 2 due to physical inactivity and obesity; the same cause as in adults (Wilson, 2013). Increasing rates of extreme obesity in children are being reported and with this alarming trend comes not only Type 2 diabetes but also other 'adult onset' diseases such as obstructive sleep apnoea (where fat around the neck impedes breathing during sleep); fatty liver disease (steatohepatitis); and heart disease, with severely obese adolescents being particularly vulnerable (Kubik, et al., 2013). In terms of the psychological effect of obesity in children, they are known to experience significant alienation; low self-esteem; body dissatisfaction; depressive symptoms; poor control of eating behaviour; harmful weight control behaviours (such as anorexia and/ or bulimia nervosa); and impaired social relationships (Vander Wal and Mitchell, 2011; Zeller, et al., 2006). A further study has assessed the health-related quality of life experienced by obese children and adolescents as being similar to that of young persons diagnosed with cancer (Schwimmer, et al., 2003). It has also been confirmed that the level of weight-related distress increases with age and is worse in girls than in boys (Erickskson, et al., 2000; French, et al., 1995).

In order to tackle the problem of childhood obesity the whole family must become involved as obesity is often related to poor nutrition and family understanding of portion control. This type of approach relies on health education about reducing calories and increasing the amount of regular exercise, benefiting the whole family (Barlow, 2007). Few studies have assessed the long-term outcome of behavioural therapy in obese young people, although Kubik, et al. (2013) have suggested that this approach is not generally successful, although when combined with weight loss medication this situation improves (Chanoine, et al., 2005). Weight loss surgery is considered for young patients with life-threatening obesity but this is only in extreme cases where the need outweighs the risk. In such cases a long-term risk assessment must be undertaken (Hsia, et al., 2012). The success rate of bariatric surgery in adolescents has been reported as being similar to that in adults, with 40–60 percent of excess weight lost in the first year and >75 percent by the end of the second year, (Kubik, et al., 2013; Hsia, et al., 2012).

Weight loss surgery in young adults has the same effect as in older individuals of resolving or significantly improving high blood pressure, insulin resistance, Type 2 diabetes and high levels of unhealthy blood fats. In terms of psychological benefit, depression, anxiety and self-perception are also improved following stomach restriction/malabsorption procedures after as little as four months (Jarvholm, et al., 2012) whilst a further study has shown that this improvement is still present after four years (Zeller, et al., 2011). This outcome shows that mental health is strongly associated with weight control although, as with the adult bariatric surgery population, psychological gains were seen in young persons who had recently had surgery but had not achieved significant weight loss, and in those who had obesity issues. This is thought to be because there is some weight change with an associated reduction in comorbid disease, or because the patient's improved self-perception renders weight issues less of a concern (Zeller, et al., 2011).

It is clear that weight loss surgery has significant physical and psychological benefits for the young and adult individuals. However, the benefit of surgery must outweigh any potential short and long-term risks as obesity is driven by eating disorders that may mean the patient has no remission of their psychological symptoms post-surgery. Because weight loss equates with a perception of control over both obesity and life issues it may be the case, as previous comments have shown, that the individual equates weight loss surgery with solving all the problems they face and that the reality is difficult to accept.

Glossary of Terms

Acrocyanosis: intolerance to cold manifesting as bluish skin discolouration on the fingers, nose and ears due to poor circulation.

Acute adrenocortical hypofunction: (also called Addison's crisis or adrenal crisis) which is a medical emergency. It occurs due to a sudden reduction in hydrocortisone.

Addison's disease: (also known as chronic cortical hypofunction or adrenocortical insufficiency) develops due to slow destruction of the adrenal cortex due to auto-immune mechanism.

ADHD: Attention Deficit Hyperactivity Disorder.

Adipokines: are produced by fat cells and are known to cause Type 2 diabetes, high blood pressure and narrowing of the arteries.

Adiponectin: hormone produced by the fat cells that causes sensitivity of tissues to insulin.

Adipose: fat tissue.

Adrenal insufficiency: an alternative name for Addison's disease. A condition where there is reduced hormone production due to auto-immune damage reducing the release of hormones such as cortisol.

Aldosterone: a hormone secreted by the adrenal glands which acts to increase the uptake of sodium and the secretion of potassium.

ALT: Alanine Transaminase.

Amygdala: the part of the brain responsible for generating negative emotions.

Androgens: sex hormones.

Anorexia nervosa: where there is an obsessive fear of gaining weight resulting in severe dietary restriction

Anterior cingulated cortex: the area of the brain responsible for attention, self-awareness and regulation.

Anti-atherogenic: medications that reduce fatty deposits in the artery walls.

Anti-hypertensive drugs: reduce blood pressure.

Anti-neoplastic drugs: prevent abnormal tissue growth.

AST: Aspartate Transaminase.

Atheroma: pertaining to atherosclerosis – fatty deposits in the arteries causing narrowing and arterial disease.

Atherosclerosis: a degenerative disease of the arteries associated with fatty deposits on the inner walls leading to reduced blood flow.

Auto-immune diseases: chronic health conditions such as Type 1 diabetes, where the disease is caused by immune system attack.

Auto-immune hepatitis: an auto-immune disorder of the liver occurring when the immune system attacks the liver cells, causing inflammation.

Bariatric surgery: weight loss surgery where a gastric band is fitted or a small pouch created by dividing the stomach so that calorie intake is drastically reduced.

Basal rate: in terms of insulin pump therapy this is the set amount of background insulin delivered per hour to maintain blood glucose levels within normal limits.

BDI: Beck Depression Inventory.

BDI: Beck Depression Inventory.

Beri beri: vitamin B1 deficiency which can be either dry (causing heart and circulatory problems), or wet (causing neurological problems accompanied by muscle weakness).

Bilopancreatic diversion: surgery to reduce the size of the stomach and intestine to limit food intake and absorption

Bolus rate: in terms of insulin pump therapy, this is the amount of insulin delivered for each meal or to correct a high blood glucose reading.

Bradycardia: slow heartbeat.

Brittle Type 1 diabetes: where Type 1 diabetes is very difficult to control due to frequent and unexplained hypo- and hyperglycaemia.

Bulimia nervosa: a disorder characterised by binge eating, then vomiting or laxative abuse.

Bupropion: an anti-depressant known to exacerbate the symptoms of psoriasis.

Calcific periarthritis: a condition where calcium deposits occur in the shoulder joints and soft tissues, restricting movement.

Cardiac tamponade: where the cardiac sac fills with blood, putting pressure on the heart.

Catabolism: chemical reactions that break down complex compounds with the release of energy.

Catecholamine: substances produced by the adrenal glands in response to stress, triggering the release of glucagon by the liver.

CBT: Cognitive Behavioural Therapy is a psychotherapeutic treatment addressing dysfunctional emotional patterns, maladaptive behaviours, and cognitive processes using goal-driven systematic methods.

Charcot joints: a chronic complication of diabetes where there is degeneration of the joints of the foot due to nerve damage, loss of sensation and excess areas of pressure.

Cheiroarthropathy: an over-production of collagen in the joints of the hands causing stiffening and limited movement.

Cholelithiasis: gallstones.

Chronic asthma: where the patient has a persistent wheeze and cough and is permanently breathless with frequent chest infections.

Chronic cortical hypofunction: an alternative name for Addison's disease.

Coeliac disease: a chronic auto-immune condition triggered by an intolerance to gluten (a protein found in cereal grains such as wheat) which cause chronic inflammation of the small bowel.

Cognition: the process of getting knowledge, including perception, intuition and reasoning.

Cognitive reappraisal: when the individual is consciously aware of their cognitions and alters them accordingly.

Collagen: the most-abundant protein in the body. It strengthens connective tissues and cushions the joints.

Colitis: a chronic condition where the colon and rectum become inflamed.

Comorbid medical conditions: conditions such as diabetes that are present in the individual at the same time as (for example) depression.

Concordance: the extent to which an individual follows a given treatment regime.

Contraindications: drug interactions.

Control Theory: the idea that goal-setting and action planning can be used to change behaviour.

Cortisol: (Hydrocortisone) a glucocorticoid hormone which maintains the level of glucose in the blood plasma.

C-peptide: an essential but biologically inactive building block of insulin formed during the manufacture of insulin by the beta cells of the pancreas.

CSII: Continuous Subcutaneous Insulin Infusion.

DAFNE: Dosage Adjustment For Normal Eating – Type 1 education.

Decisional balance: weighing up the pros and cons of changing health behaviour.

DESMOND: Diabetes Education and Self-Management for Ongoing and Newly Diagnosed.

Diabetes Insipidus: a rare condition affecting the pituitary gland, characterised by severe thirst and frequent urination that does not contain glucose.

Diabetic ketoacidosis (DKA): is a medical emergency where there is severe disruption of the body's acidity balance due to prolonged hyperglycaemia.

Diabulimia: is the deliberate under-dosing or omission of insulin to achieve rapid weight loss by inducing hyperglycaemia and ketoacidosis. It is common in females with Type 1 diabetes.

Disordered eating: describes a range of eating-related problems, from dieting to anorexia and bulimia.

Dyslipidaemia: a disorder of fat metabolism including lipoprotein under- or over-production, often manifesting as high blood cholesterol.

Dysthyroid optic neuropathy: a rare sight-threatening condition associated with Graves' disease (over-production of thyroid hormones) causing compression of the optic nerve.

Duodenum: the first part of the small intestine.

Eating disorders: are psychological illnesses marked by disturbed eating behaviour, distorted food intake, disordered attitudes to eating, and inadequate methods of weight control.

ECT: electro-convulsive therapy.

Empowerment: increasing the individual's understanding of their diabetes and potential for self-care so that an informed choice can be made.

Exenatide: a blood glucose-lowering medication used to treat Type 2 diabetes, known to reduce itching in psoriasis.

Expressive repression: having awareness of cognitions and altering them accordingly.

External locus of control: a term describing individuals who do not feel as though they have any control over what happens to them because their lives are dictated by or subject to other people's actions.

Extrinsic asthma: where external factors (allergens) such as smoke, pollen, dust etc. trigger an attack.

Fluoxetine: an anti-depressant suitable for the treatment of depression in people with diabetes, but shown in some studies to exacerbate symptoms of psoriasis.

Folic acid: a water-soluble vitamin also known as vitamin B9.

FSH: Follicle Stimulating Hormone.

Gastroparesis: delayed emptying of the stomach causing bloating, early fullness and rarely, upper quadrant pain. The condition also occurs in people with diabetes due to autonomic nerve damage.

GI: Gastrointestinal.

Glucagon: attaches to the liver cells to make them release stored glucose quickly.

Glucocorticoid disruption: the release of hormones, such as cortisol, in times of stress.

Glucocorticoid hormones: are mainly cortisol and adrenocorticotropic hormone which are released during times of stress.

Gluconeogenesis: the metabolic pathway resulting in the generation of glucose from non-carbohydrate sources, e.g. amino acids, glycerol or lactic acid enabling the release of glucose into the body.

Gluten: a protein found in cereal grains such as wheat, added to bread to make it rise.

Glycosylation: the breakdown of proteins into glucose.

GnTR: Gonadotrophin-releasing hormone.

Graves' disease: a condition describing the production of too much thyroxin by the thyroid gland.

Hashimoto's thyroiditis: also known as Chronic Lymphocytic Thyroiditis where auto-immune attack leads to too little thyroxin being produced.

HbA1c (glycosylated haemoglobin): blood test to measure the amount of glucose sticking to the red blood cells over a three-month period.

HbA1c (glycosylated haemoglobin): blood test to measure the amount of glucose sticking to the red blood cells over a three-month period.

HBM: Health Belief Model.

HDL: High Density Lipids.

Hippocampus: the part of the brain responsible for consolidating memory.

Hyperglycaemia: high blood glucose levels >15.0 mmol/L.

Hyperleptinaemia: high levels of leptin, a hormone involved in regulation of body fat, hunger and feeling full after meals,

Hyperlipidaemia: an increased level of harmful fats in the blood.

Hypertension: high blood pressure.

Hyperthyroidism: over-production of thyroid hormones.

Hypoglycaemia: low blood glucose levels <3.5 mmol/L

Hypotension: low blood pressure.

Hypothalamic amenorrhea syndrome: absence of menstruation due to anorexia.

Hypothalamus: a region of the brain situated below the thalamus, coordinating the autonomic nervous system and the activity of the pituitary gland to regulate body temperature, hunger, thirst, sleep and emotional activity.

Hypothermia: a reduced body temperature below 35 degrees centigrade.

Hypothyroidism: under-production of thyroid hormones.

Immunosuppressant drugs: prevent organ rejection after transplant surgery by preventing immune system attack.

Incidence: the number of new cases of a disease that develop in a population.

Insula: part of the brain that is crucial to understanding what it feels like to be human. The starting place of social emotions such as guilt, atonement, moral intuition, empathy, and emotional response to music.

Insulin resistance: where the pancreas produces more insulin to lower raised blood glucose levels in pre-diabetes or untreated Type 2 diabetes because the action of insulin on the cells is impaired by the presence of fat.

Interleukin-6: a substance associated with glucose intolerance that increases the inflammatory response of the immune system in severe illness.

Internalising: having an internal rather than an external locus of control.

Internal locus of control: a term describing individuals who perceive they have control over what happens to them because their decisions and actions are self-determined.

Internalising: having an internal rather than an external locus of control.

Intrinsic asthma: where there is no apparent external cause. Asthma can be episodic, where attacks occurs at any time for a variable length and severity.

Iodide: iodine removed from the blood and combined with proteins in the thyroid gland to produce the hormone thyroxin.

Islet cell antibodies: proteins in the blood which destroy the insulin-producing beta cells of the pancreas.

Jejunum: the second part of the small intestine.

Ketoacidosis: an acute and significant complication of Type 1 diabetes that occurs when the blood glucose level becomes consistently very high

(>15mmol/L or >270mg/dl) causing the breakdown of fats as an alternative source of energy to glucose that cannot be easily used in the lack of insulin.

Lactate: a salt of lactic acid.

Lanugo: fine downy hair growth on the sides of the face and down the spine, associated with anorexia nervosa.

Laparoscopic: gastric surgery performed via a small incision in the abdomen.

Laparoscopic sleeve gastrectomy: surgery where a small portion of the stomach is sectioned off so that it takes less food to become full.

Lap band surgery: insertion of an adjustable gastric band.

Learned helplessness: a state where an individual feels they can do nothing about a situation and they become stressed, depressed, anxious and often hostile, losing their initiative as a result.

Leptin: a hormone made by fat cells that is involved in the regulation of body fat.

Leukopenia: anaemia and a low white blood cell count.

LH: Luteinising Hormone.

Lipolysis: the regulation of protein synthesis and the mobilisation of fat controlled by growth hormone.

Liraglutide: a blood glucose-lowering medication used to treat Type 2 diabetes, known to reduce itching in psoriasis.

Lithium: an anti-depressant known to exacerbate the symptoms of psoriasis.

Macrophages: cells that remove bacteria and debris from the blood stream and tissues.

Macrovascular: pertaining to the large blood vessels.

MBCT: Mindfulness-Based Cognitive Therapy.

MDI: multiple daily injections.

Metabolic syndrome: a group of pathophysiological states and cardiac risk factors which includes abdominal obesity, impaired glucose regulation, high blood fats, reduced high-density lipids, and hypertension. Insulin resistance means that glucose absorption by cells stimulated by insulin is reduced.

Microvascular: pertaining to the capillaries and small blood vessels.

Models: an example of patterns people may wish to follow.

MOI: Monoaminine Oxidase Inhibitor.

Morbidity: the state of being diseased; the morbidity rate being expressed as the number of cases of disease occurring within a particular number of the population.

Mortality: The number of deaths in a given period or from a given cause.

Motivation: is defined in psychological terms as consisting of internal processes that spur us on to satisfy some need.

Motivational interviewing: a patient-centred technique designed to prepare an individual for behavioural change, also called brief negotiation.

Myocardial infarction: destruction of a portion of the myocardium of the heart due to poor or absent blood supply.

Nephropathy: is a chronic complication of diabetes caused by persistently high blood glucose levels leading to hardening of the kidney tissue and changes in the structure of the tubular epithelial cells of the kidneys

Neurons: brain cells.

Neuropathy: is a complex condition where nerve damage occurs, especially in the feet and hands.

Neuroplasticity: changing the way one thinks to enable the growth of new neuron connections in the brain.

Normoglycaemia: a normal level of blood glucose within acceptable limits of 4.0–7.0 mmol/L.

Obesity: a body mass index of above 30 kg/m^2

Osteoarthritis: a very common condition in the elderly due to wear and tear of the bones and joints (most commonly the weight-bearing knees and hips), and in younger people this develops in bone following trauma

Osteoarthropathy: a condition seen in people with Type 2 diabetes affecting the weight-bearing bones of the feet.

Osteopenia: a lack of bone density.

Osteoporosis: brittleness of the bones caused by lack of calcium.

Outcome expectancy: the expected results of diabetes self-management behaviour.

Orthostatic hypotension: low blood pressure.

Oxidative stress: cell breakdown where they die or are damaged beyond repair.

Peptides: small organic compounds made up of two or more amino acids.

Pericardial effusion: a collection of fluid in the pericardial sac surrounding the heart.

Peripheral neuropathy: a chronic complication of diabetes which occurs in two forms: diffuse neuropathy, commonly appearing as disorders of sensation in the extremities of the body; and distal polyneuropathy, affecting many nerves of the hands and feet.

Pessimistic attribution styles: consistently blaming oneself for negative things that happen and displaying passive (emotionally-focussed) rather than proactive coping strategies.

PET: Positron Emission Tomography.

Pneumoperineum: air in the abdominal cavity.

Pneumothorax: air in the pleural space causing the lung to collapse.

Post-prandial: after meals.

Pre-diabetes: (also known as insulin resistance) where blood glucose levels are higher than normal but lower than established thresholds for diabetes itself.

Prevalence: refers to the pattern of occurrence of a disease.

Primary biliary cirrhosis: is an auto-immune disease of the liver where there is slow progressive destruction of the bile ducts causing bile and other toxins to build up in the liver, causing scarring and cirrhosis.

Primary sclerosing cholangitis: a disease of the bile ducts causing inflammation and obliterative fibrosis of the bile ducts inside and outside the liver leading to liver failure and potentially bile duct and liver cancer.

Proactive consideration: when the individual considers the effect of a new behaviour.

Pro-insulin: the molecule of which insulin is made by the beta cells of the pancreas.

Psoriasis: an auto-immune skin condition causing red, flaky, crusty patches covered with silvery scales appearing on the elbows, knees, scalp and lower back. These can become itchy and sore.

Pulmonary embolus: blockage of the pulmonary artery, or a branch of it, by a blood clot usually originating in the leg. Large pulmonary emboli can be fatal.

Purging behaviour: is classified as self-induced vomiting and laxative abuse which occurs at least twice a week for a period of three months.

Reactive hypoglycaemia: a reduction in blood glucose level due to the body producing too much insulin.

Regulation: appropriately-managed diabetes.

Resistin: a substance released by the fat cells that 'resists' the action of insulin on the cells, preventing the lowering of blood glucose.

Retinopathy: is a chronic complication of diabetes which describes a number of symptoms including abnormal dilation of the blood vessels of the eyes and haemorrhages of the retina. In advanced cases the retina becomes heavily scarred and this may lead to blindness.

Self-efficacy: the individual's belief that they have the ability to achieve the desired effect of effective diabetes self-management.

Self-gratification: satisfaction.

Self-reactive influences: sensitivities.

Self-regulation theory: suggests that the individual reflects on their progress and feeds this information back to the health professionals providing their care because it can help to maintain a behaviour change. However, this reflection of outcomes and focus on the need to achieve an improvement may actually be de-motivating.

Serotonin: a hormone that gives us a sense of wellbeing. It acts as a neuro-transmitter to relay signals from one area of the brain to another.

Severe hypoglycaemia: disabling low blood glucose levels requiring the assistance of another person.

Sickness behaviour: as a co-ordinated set of behaviour changes that develop in all cases of illness and include low motivation to eat, listlessness, fatigue, malaise, a reduced interest in social activity, a change in sleep patterns, an inability to experience pleasure, an exaggerated response to pain and a lack of concentration.

Sleep apnoea: where fat around the neck impedes breathing during sleep.

SLT: Social Learning Theory.

SMAS: Super Mesenteric Artery Syndrome, where the duodenum is compressed between the spine and the aorta.

SNRIs: Selective Noradrenaline Reuptake Inhibitors – an anti-depressant medication.

SOC: Stages of Change model.

Sorbitol: a substance metabolised from excessive glucose which triggers chronic diabetes complications as the large sorbitol molecules damages cells.

SSRIs: Selective Serotonin Reuptake Inhibitors – an anti-depressant medication.

Status asthmaticus: where an asthma attack is severe and lasts for more than 24 hours with no response to medication, leading to increased heart rate and potential lack of conciseness.

Steatohepatitis: fatty liver disease.

Steatosis: an increase in liver enzymes associated with the intravenous feeding of dextrose to patients with anorexia.

Stricture: the growth of scar tissue following surgery of injury resulting in narrowing, e.g. intestinal stricture following bariatric surgery.

Systemic conditions: having an effect on the whole body (such as diabetes).

Tension pneumothorax: where a valve develops in the lung allowing air to escape into the pleural space which cannot escape, pushing the heart, lungs, trachea, oesophagus and other structures towards the unaffected lung.

TCA: tricyclic anti-depressants.

T-cells: thymus lymphocytes which circulate in the blood and lymphatic fluid to trigger the immune system to fight an infection.

Thalamus: the relay station of the brain.

The hygiene hypothesis: proposes that infections in early childhood may reduce the risk of allergic diseases by strengthening the immune system's defence.

Thrombopenia: a low red blood cell count.

Thyrotoxicosis: the over production of thyroid hormones by the thyroid gland due to the gland itself, or due to ineffective storage or leakage of the hormones.

TRA: Theory of Reasoned Action.

Trachea: windpipe.

Transaminases: enzymes produced by the liver which break down amino acids and convert them to energy storage molecules.

TSH: Thyroid Stimulating Hormone.

Vasoconstriction of the arteries: narrowing.

Vasodilation of the arteries: widening.

Wernick'e encephalopathy: a neurological disorder caused by vitamin B1 (thiamine) deficiency.

References

Abella, E., Feliu, E., Granada, I. (2002) Bone marrow changes in anorexia nervosa are correlated with the amount of weight loss and not with other clinical findings. *American Journal of Clinical Pathology* 118: 582–588.

Abid, N., Mcglone, O., Cardwell, C., et al. (2011) Clinical and metabolic effects of gluten free diet in children with type 1 diabetes and coeliac disease. *Pediatric Diabetes* 12(4): part 1, 322–325.

Abiles, V., Rodrıguez-Ruiz, S., Abiles, J., et al. (2010) Psychological characteristics of morbidly obese candidates for bariatric surgery. *Obesity Surgery* 20(2): 161–167.

Abrams, R. (1988) *Electroconvulsive Therapy*. Oxford: Oxford University Press.

Abramson, J., Berger, A., Krumholz, H.M., et al. (2001) Depression and risk of heart failure among older persons with isolated systolic hypertension. *Archive of Internal Medicine* 161(14): 1725–1730.

Ackard, D.M., Neumark-Sztainer, V.N., Schmitz, K.H., et al. (2008) Disordered eating and body dissatisfaction in adolescents with Type 1 diabetes and a population-based comparison sample: comparative prevalence and clinical implications. *Pediatric Diabetes* 9: 312–319.

Adams, T.D., Gress, R.E., Smith, S.C., et al. (2007) Long-term mortality after gastric bypass surgery. *New England Journal of Medicine* 357: 753–761.

Affenito, S.G. & Adams, C.H. (2001) Are eating disorders more prevalent in females with Type 1 diabetes mellitus when the impact of insulin omission is considered? *Nutrition Review* 59: 179–182.

Aggarwal, S., Lebwohl, B., Green, P.H.R. (2012) Screening for celiac disease in average-risk and high-risk populations. *Therapeutic Advances in Gastroenterology* 5(1): 37–47.

Ahmad, L.A. & Crandall, J.P. (2010) Type 2 diabetes prevention: a review. *Clinical Diabetes* 28(2): 53–58.

Aikens, J.E. (2010) Prospective associations between emotional distress and poor outcomes in type 2 diabetes. *Diabetes Care* 35: 2472–2478.

Al'Abadie, M.S., Kent, G.G., Gawkrodger, D.J. (1994) The relationship between stress and the onset and exacerbation of psoriasis and other skin conditions. *British Journal of Dermatology* 130: 199–203.

Al-Arouj, A., Khalil, A., Buse, J., et al. (2010) Recommendations for management of diabetes during Ramadan. *Diabetes Care* 33(10): 1895–1904.

Aliyu, I. (2014) Acute psychosis following diabetic ketoacidosis in an 11-year-old: management challenges in a resource-limited setting. *Sudan Medical Monitor* 9(2) http://www.sudanmedicalmonitor.org

Aljahlan, M., Lee, K.C., Toth, E. (1999) Limited joint mobility in diabetes. *Postgraduate Medicine* 105(2): 99–106.

Alpsoy, E., Ozcan, E., Cetin, L., et al. (1998) Is the efficacy of topical corticosteroid therapy for psoriasis vulgaris enhanced by concurrent moclobemide therapy? A double-blind, placebo-controlled study. Journal of the American Academic Dermatology 38: 197–200.

Alves, C., Diniz, A.B., Souza, M.B., et al. (2007) Controversies in the association between type 1 diabetes and asthma. *Arquivos Brasileiros de Endocrinol & Metabologia* 51: 930–937.

American Diabetes Association (2012) Diagnosis and classification of diabetes mellitus. *Diabetes Care* 35: S64–71.

American Psychiatric Association (2013) *Diagnostic Statistical Manual of Mental Disorders.* 5th edition, Washington DC: American Psychiatric Association.

American Psychiatric Association (2006) *Practice Guideline for the Treatment of Patients with Eating Disorders.* 3rd edition. http://www.psych.org/psych_pract

Anderson, R. (2008) New MRC guidance on evaluating complex interventions. *British Medical Journal* 337: a1937.

Anderson, R.J., Grigsby, A.B., Freedland, K.E., et al. (2002) Anxiety and poor glycemic control: a meta-analytic review of the literature. *International Journal of Psychiatry and Medicine* 32: 235–247.

Anderson, R.J., Freedland, K.E., Clouse, R.E., et al. (2001) The prevalence of comorbid depression in adults with diabetes: a meta-analysis. *Diabetes Care* 24: 1069–1078.

Anderson, R.M., Funnell, M.M., Fitzgerald, T.J., et al. (2000) The Diabetes Empowerment Scale: a measure of psychosocial self-efficacy. *Diabetes Care* 23(6): 739–743.

Ansaldi, N., Palmas, T., Corrias, A., et al. (2003) Autoimmune thyroid disease and celiac disease in children. *Journal of Pediatric Gastroenterology and Nutrition* 37(1): 63–66.

Ajzen, I. (1985) From intentions to action: a theory of planned behaviour. In: Kuhl. J., Beckman, J. (Eds.), *Action Control: From Cognition to Behaviour.* Springer-Verlag: Berlin.

Ajzen, I. & Fishbein, M. (1975) *Belief, Attitude, Intention and Behaviour: An introduction to Theory and Research.* Addison-Wesley: Reading, Massachusetts.

Arkkila, P.E., Kantola, I.M., Vikkari, J.S. (1997) Limited joint mobility in non-insulin-dependent diabetic patients: correlation to control of diabetes, atherosclerotic vascular disease, and other diabetic complications. *Journal of Diabetes Complications* 11(4): 208–217.

Arkkila, P.E., Kantola, I.M., Vikkari, J.S. (1994) Limited joint movement in type 1 diabetic patients: correlation to other complications. *Journal of Internal Medicine* 236(2): 215–216.

Arnold, M., Butler, P., Anderson, R., et al. (1995) Guideline for facilitating a patient empowerment programme. *The Diabetes Educator* 21(4): 308–312.

Aronson, D. (2008) Hyperglycemia and the pathobiology of diabetic complications. *Advanced Cardiology* 45: 1–16.

Aspinwall, L.G. & Tedeschi, R. (2010) The value of positive psychology for health psychology: progress and pitfalls in examining the relationship of positive phenomenon to health. *Annals of Behavioural Medicine* 39(1): 4–15.

Asvoid, B.O., Sandt, T., Hestad, K., et al. (2010) Cognitive function in Type 1 diabetes with early exposure to severe hypoglycaemia. *Diabetes Care* 33: 1945–1947.

Auer, R.N. (2004a) Hypoglycaemic brain damage. *Metabolic Brain Disease* 19: 169–175.

Auer, R.N. (2004b) Hypoglycaemic brain damage. *Forensic Science International* 146: 105–110.

Austin, A.J. & Dearey, I.J. (1999) Effect of repeated hypoglycaemia on cognitive function. *Diabetes Care* 22: 1273–1277.

Avenell, A., Sattar, N., Lean, M. (2006) Management: Part I, behaviour change, diet and activity. *British Medical Journal* 740–750.

Ayturk, S., Gursoy, A., Kut, A., et al. (2009) Metabolic syndrome and its components are associated with increased thyroid volume and nodule prevalence in a mild-to-moderate iodine-deficient area. *European Journal of Endocrinology* 161(4): 599–605.

Azizi, F. (2002) Research in Islamic fasting and health. *Annuls of Saudi Medicine* 22:186–191.

Babyak, M., Blumenthal, J.A., Herman, S., et al. (2000) Exercise treatment for major depression: maintenance of therapeutic benefit at 10 months. *Psychosomatic Medicine* 62(5): 633–638.

Baker, R.A., Pikalov, A., Tran, Q.V., et al. (2009) Atypical antipsychotic drugs and diabetes mellitus in the US Food andDrug Administration Adverse Event database: A systematic Bayesian signal detection analysis. *Psychopharmacology Bulletin* 42: 11–31.

Bakker, S.F., Tushuizen, M.E., Stokvis-Brantsma, W.H.S., et al. (2013a) Frequent delay of coeliac disease diagnosis in symptomatic patients with type 1 diabetes mellitus: clinical and genetic characteristics. *European Journal of Internal Medicine* 24(5): 456–460.

Bakker, S.F., Tushuizen, M.E., von Blomberg, M.E., et al. (2013b) Type 1 diabetes and celiac disease in adults: glycemic control and diabetic complications. *Acta Diabetologica*, 50(3): 319–324.

Balci, A., Balci, D.D., Yonden, Z., et al. (2010) Increased amount of visceral fat in patients with psoriasis contributes to metabolic syndrome. *Dermatology* 220: 32–37.

Bandura, A. (2001) Social cognitive theory: an agentic perspective. *Annual Review of Psychology* 52: 1–26.

Bandura, A. (2000) Health promotion from the perspective of social cognitive theory. In: Norman P, Abraham C, Conner M (Eds) *Understanding and Changing Health Behaviour: From Health Beliefs to Self-Regulation.* Harwood Academic: Amsterdam.

Bandura, A. (1999a) Moral disengagement in the perpetration of inhumanities. *Perspectives of Social Psychology Review* 3: 193–209.

Bandura, A. (1999b) Social Cognitive Theory: An Agentic Perspective. *Asian Journal of Social Psychology* 2: 21–41.

Bandura, A. (1991) Social cognitive theory of self-regulation. *Theories of Cognitive Self-Regulation* 50: 248-287.

Bandura, A. (1977a) *Social Learning Theory.* Prentice Hall: New Jersey, USA.

Bandura, A. (1977b) Self-efficacy: towards a unifying theory of behaviour change. *Psychological Review* 84: 191–215.

Bao, F., Yu, L., Babuetal, S. (1999) One third of HLADQ2 homozygous patients with type 1 diabetes express celiac disease-associated transglutaminase autoantibodies. *Journal of Autoimmunity* 13(1): 143–148.

Bardella, M.T., Vecchi, M., Conte, D., et al. (1999) Chronic unexplained hypertransaminasemia may be caused by occult celiac disease. *Hepatology* 29(3): 654–657.

Bardella, M.T., Fraquelli, M., Quatrini, M., et al. (1995) Prevalence of hypertransaminasemia in adult celiac patients and effect of gluten-free diet. *Hepatology* 22(3): 833–836.

Barker, J.M., Yu, J., Yu, L., et al. (2005) Autoantibody "subspecificity" in type 1 diabetes: risk for organ-specific autoimmunity clusters in distinct groups. *Diabetes Care* 28(4): 850–855.

Barlow, S.E. (2007) Expert committee recommendations regarding the prevention, assessment, and treatment of child and adolescent over-weight and obesity: summary report. *Pediatrics* 120: S164–192.

Barnett, A.H. & Grice, J. (2011) *New Mechanisms in Glucose Control.* Chichester, West Sussex: John Wiley & Co. Limited.

Barry, M.J. & Edgman-Levitan, S. (2012) Shared decision-making – the pinnacle of PC care. *Emergency Medicine* 366: 780–781.

Basavaraj, K.H., Ashok, N.M., Rashmi, R., et al. (2010) The role of drugs in the induction and/or exacerbation of psoriasis. *International Journal of Dermatology* 49: 1351–1361.

Battaglia, M.R., Alemzadeh, R., Katte, H., et al. (2006) Brief report: disordered eating & psychological factors in adolescent females with Type 1 diabetes mellitus. *Journal of Pediatric Psychology* 31: 552–556.

Baumeister, H., Hutter, N., Bengel, J. (2012) Psychological and pharmacological interventions for depression in patients with diabetes mellitus and depression. *Cochrane Database Systematic Review* 12.

Baumeister, R.F. & Tierney, J. (2012) Willpower: Rediscovering the Greatest Human Strength. USA: Random House, Penguin Press.

Baumeister, R.F. (2003) Ego depletion and self-regulation failure: a resource model of self-control. *Alcohol Clinical Expertise and Research* 27: 281–284.

BBC (15th August 2015a) Diabetes increases 60% in 10 years. www.bbc.co.uk

BBC (26th August 2015b) Diabetes is responsible for 22,000 extra deaths. www.bbc.co.uk

Bech, K., Damsbo, P., Eldrup, E., et al. (1996) β-Cell function and glucose and lipid oxidation in Graves' disease. *Clinical Endocrinology* 44(1): 59–66.

Beck, A.T., Rush, A.J., Shaw, B.F., et al. (1979) *Cognitive Therapy of Depression.* New York: Guilford Press.

Beck, A.T. & Beamesderfer, A. (1974) Assessment of depression: the depression inventory. *Modern problems of Pharmacopsychiatry* 7: 151–169.

Becker, M.H. & Janz, N.K. (1985) The health belief model applied to understanding diabetes regime compliance. *The Diabetes Educator* 11: 41–47.

Becker, M.H. (1974) *The Health Belief Model and Personal Health Behaviour.* London, England: Charles B. Slack, Thoroughfare.

Beer, S.F., Parr, J.H., Temple, R.C., et al. (1989) The effect of thyroid disease on proinsulin and C-peptide levels. *Clinical Endocrinology* 30(4): 379–383.

Behre, H.M., Kliesch, S., Leifke, E. (1997) Long-term effect of testosterone therapy on bone mineral density in hypogonadal men. *Journal of Clinical Endocrinology Metabolism* 82: 2386–2390.

Benchimol, E.I., Manuel, D.G., To, T., et al. (2015) Asthma, Type 1 and Type 2 diabetes mellitus and inflammatory bowel disease among South Asian Immigrants to Canada and their children: a population-based cohort study. *PLoS One* 10(4): e0123599.

Bener, A, Ghuloum, S., Al-Hamaq, A.O., et al. (2012) Association between psychological distress and gastrointestinal symptoms in diabetes mellitus. *World Journal of Diabetes* 3: 123–129.

Berger, J.R. (2004) The neurological complications of bariatric surgery. *Archive of Neurology* 61: 1185–1189.

Bermudez, O. & Sommer, J. (2012) Beyond "diabulimia": the dual diagnosis of eating disorder and diabetes. *The Pulse* 31(2): 9–12.

Betterle, C., Lazzaratto, F., Spadaccino, A.C., et al. (2006) Celiac disease in North Italian patients with autoimmune Addison's disease. *European Journal of Endocrinology,* 154(2): 275–279.

Bhattacharyya, A. & Wiles, P.G. (1999) Diabetic ketoacidosis precipitated by thyrotoxicosis. *Postgraduate Medical Journal* 75 (883): 291–292.

Biagi, F., Campanella, J., Soriani, A., et al. (2006) Prevalence of coeliac disease in Italian patients affected by Addison's disease. *Scandinavian Journal of Gastroenterology* 41 (3): 302–305.

Biddle, S.J., Fox, K.R., Boutcher, S.H. (Eds.) (2000) *Physical Activity and Psychological Well-Being.* New York: Routledge.

Biffl, W.L., Narayanan, V., Gaudiani, J.L., et al. (2010) The management of pneumothorax in patients with anorexia nervosa: A case report and review of the literature. *Patient Safety in Surgery* 4: 1.

Bild, D.E., Selby, J.V., Sinnock, P., et al. (1989) Lower-extremity amputation in people with diabetes. Epidemiology and prevention. *Diabetes Care* 12: 24–31.

Bishop, G.D., Smelser, N.J., Baltes, P.B. (2001) *Emotions and Health.* Oxford: Pergamon.

Black, M.H., Anderson, A., Bell, R.A., et al. (2011) Prevalence of asthma and its association with glycemic control among youth with diabetes. *Pediatrics* 128: e839–e847.

Blakeslee, S. (2007) A small part of the brain, and its profound effects. *New York Times,* 6th February.

Bluestone, J.A., Buckner, J.H., Fitch, M., et al. (2015) Type 1 diabetes immunotherapy using polyclonal regulatory T cells. *Science Translational Medicine* 7(315): 315ra189.

Blumenthal, J.A., Babyak, M.A., Moore, K.A., et al. (1999) Effects of exercise training on older patients with major depression. *Archive of Internal Medicine* 159(19): 2349–2356.

Bocchieri, L.E., Meana, M., Fisher, B.L. (2002) A review of psychosocial outcomes of surgery for morbid obesity. *Journal of Psychosomatic Research* 52(3): 155–165.

Boden, G., Sargrad, K., Homko, C., et al. (2005) Effect of a low-carbohydrate diet on appetite, blood glucose levels and insulin resistance in obese patients with Type 2 diabetes. *Annals of Internal Medicine* 142: 403–411.

Boden, G. & Hoeldtke, R.D. (2003) Nerves, fat, and insulin resistance. *New England Journal of Medicine* 349: 1966–1967.

Boehncke, S., Thaci, D., Beschmann, H., et al. (2007) Psoriasis patients show signs of insulin resistance. *British Journal of Dermatology* 157: 1249–1251.

Boehncke, W., Boehncke, S., Tobin, A.M. (2011) The 'psoriatic march': a concept of how severe psoriasis may drive cardiovascular comorbidity. *Experimental Dermatology* 20: 303–307.

Boehncke, W.H., Boehncke, S., Buerger, C. (2012) Beyond immunopathogenesis. Insulin resistance and "epidermal dysfunction" *Der Hautarzt* 63:178-83.

Boule, N.G., Haddad, E., Kenny, G.P., et al. (2001) Effects of exercise on glycemic control and body mass in type 2 diabetes mellitus: a meta-analysis of controlled clinical trials. *Journal of the American Medical Association* 286 (10): 1218–1227.

Bradley, C. (1995) *Handbook of Psychology and Diabetes.* Switzerland: Churchill, Harwood Academic Publishers.

Bradley, M.M. & Lang, P.J. (2000) Measuring emotion: Behavior, feeling, and physiology. In: Nadel, R.D.L.L. (Ed.) *Cognitive Neuroscience of Emotion.* New York: Oxford University Press.

Bradshaw, B.G., Richardson, G.E., Kulkarni, K. (2007a) Thriving with diabetes: an introduction to the resiliency approach for diabetes educators. *Diabetes Educator* 33: 643–649.

Bradshaw, B.G., Richardson, G.E., Kumpfer, K., et al. (2007b) Determining the efficacy of a resiliency training approach in adults with type 2 diabetes. *Diabetes Educator* 33: 650–659.

Brauchli, Y.B., Jick, S.S., Meier, C.R. (2008) Psoriasis and the risk of incident diabetes mellitus: a population-based study. *British Journal of Dermatology* 159:1331–1337.

Bree, A.J., Puente, E.C., Dorit, D-L., et al. (2009) Diabetes increases brain damage caused by severe hypoglycaemia. *American Journal of Physiology, Endocrinology and Metabolism* 297: E194–E201.

Brehm, J.W. (1999) The intensity of emotion. *Perspective Sociology and Psychology Review* 3: 2–22.

Bremmer, S., Van Voorhees, A.S., Hsu, S., et al. (2010) Obesity and psoriasis: from the Medical Board of the National Psoriasis Foundation. *Journal of the American Academy of Dermatology* 63:1058–1069.

Broman, C.L. (1995) Leisure-time physical activity in an Afro-American population. *Journal of Behavioural Medicine* 18: 341–352.

Broome, A. & Llewelyn, S. (1995) *Health Psychology: Process and Application.* London: Chapman and Hall.

Brown, A.F., Mangione, C.M., Saliba, D., et al. (2003) Guidelines for improving the care of the older person with diabetes mellitus. *Journal of American Geriatric Society* 51: S265–S280.

Brown, C. & Mehler, P.S. (2014) Anorexia nervosa complicated by diabetes mellitus: The case for permissive hyperglycemia. *International Journal of Eating Disorders* 47: 671–674.

Brown, L.C., Newman, S.C., Majumdar, S.R., et al. (2005) Depression increased risk of Type 2 diabetes in young adults. *Diabetes Care* 28: 1063–1067.

Brown, R.F., Bartrop, R., Beaumont, P., et al. (2005) Bacterial infections in anorexia nervosa: delayed recognition increases complications. *International Journal of Eating Disorders* 37: 261–265.

Brown, S.A. & Sharpless, S.L. (2004) Osteoporosis: An under-appreciated complication of diabetes. *Clinical Diabetes* 22(1): 10–21.

Brownlee, M. & Hirsch, I.B. (2006) Glycemic variability: a hemoglobin A1c-independent risk factor for diabetic complications. *Journal of the American Medical Association* 295: 1707–1708.

Buchwald, H., Estok, R., Fahrbach, K., et al. (2009) Weight and type 2 diabetes after bariatric surgery: systematic review and meta-analysis. *American Journal of Medicine* 122: 248–256, e5.

Buchwald, H. (2005) Health implications of bariatric surgery. *Journal of the American College of Surgery* 200: 593–604

Buchwald, H., Avidor, Y., Brau, E., et al. (2004) Bariatric surgery: a systematic review and meta-analysis. *Journal of the American Medical Association* 292(14): 1724–1737.

Bulik, C.M., Hoffman, E.R., Von Holle, R. (2010) Unplanned pregnancy in women with anorexia nervosa. *Obstetrics & Gynaecology* 116: 1136–1140.

Bulik, C.M., Sullivan, P.F., Fear, J.L. (1999) Fertility and reproduction in women with anorexia nervosa: a controlled study. *Journal of Clinical Psychiatry* 60:130–135.

Burke, B.L., Arkowitz, H., Dunn, C. (2002) The efficacy of motivational interviewing and its adaptations: what we know so far. In: Miller, W.R., Rollnick, S. (Eds.) *Motivational Interviewing: Preparing People for Change*, Second Edition. New York, London: The Guilford Press.

Burns, R.B. (2001) *Essential Psychology*, Second edition. Dordrecht, The Netherlands: Kluwer Academic Publishers.

Butland, B., Jebb, S., Kopelman, P., et al. (2007) *Foresight. Tackling Obesities: Future Choices Project report*. London: Government Office for Science, Department of Innovation, Universities and Skills.

Callahan, C.M., Hui, S.L., Nienaber, N.A., et al. (1994) Longitudinal study of depression and health services use among elderly primary care patients. *Journal of the American Geriatric Society* 42: 833–838.

Camarca, M.E., Mozzillo, E., Nugnes, R., et al. (2012) Celiac disease in type 1 diabetes mellitus. *Italian Journal of Pediatrics* 38, article 10.

Camacho, T.C., Roberts, R.E., Lazarus, N.B., et al. (1991) Physical activity and depression: evidence from the Alameda County Study. *American Journal of Epidemiology* 134(2):220–231.

Carney, R.M. & Freedland, K.E. (2003) Depression, mortality, and medical morbidity in patients with coronary heart disease. *Biological Psychiatry* 54: 241–247.

Carthenon, M.R., Kinder, L.S., Fair, J.M., et al. (2003) Symptoms of depression as a risk factor for incident diabetes: findings from the National Health and Nutrition Examination Epidemiologic Follow-up Study, 1971-1992. *American Journal of Epidemiology* 158(5): 416–423.

Castaneda, C., Layne, J.E., Munoz-Orians, L., et al. (2002): A randomized controlled trial of resistance exercise training to improve glycemic control in older adults with type 2 diabetes. *Diabetes Care* 25: 2335–2341.

Cataldo, F. & Marino, V. (2003) Increased prevalence of autoimmune diseases in first-degree relatives of patients with celiac disease. *Journal of Pediatric Gastroenterology and Nutrition* 36 (4): 470–473.

Center for Disease Control and Prevention (2011) *National Diabetes Factsheet.* Atlanta, Georgia: Centre for Disease Control and Prevention.

Center for Disease Control and Prevention (2007) National Diabetes Factsheet. Atlanta, Georgia. U.S. Department of Health and Human Services; http://www.cdc.gov/Diabetes/pubs/factsheet07.htm

Cerutti, F., Bruno, G., Chiarelli, F., et al. (2004) Younger age at onset and sex predict celiac disease in children and adolescents with type 1 diabetes: an Italian multicenter study. *Diabetes Care* 27(6): 1294–1298.

Cettour-Rose, P., Theander-Carrillo, C., Asensio, C., et al. (2005) Hypothyroidism in rats decreases peripheral glucose utilisation, a defect partially corrected by central leptin infusion. *Diabetologia* 48(4): 624–633.

Chan, R., Brooks, R., Erlich, J., et al. (2009) The effects of kidney-disease-related loss on long-term dialysis patients' depression and quality of life: positive affect as a mediator. *Clinical Journal of the American Society of Nephrology* 4: 160–167.

Chanoine, J.P., Hampl, S., Jensen, C., et al. (2005) Effect of orlistat on weight and body composition in obese adolescents: a randomized controlled trial. *Journal of the American Medical Association* 293(23): 2873–2883.

Chapman, D.P., Perry, G.S., Strine, T.W. (20005) The vital link between chronic disease and depressive disorders. *Preventing Chronic Disease* 2(1): A14. http://www.cdc.gov/pcd/issues/2005/

Chatterjee, J.S. (2006) From compliance to concordance in diabetes. *Journal of Medical Ethics* 32(9): 507–510.

Chen, H.S., Wu, T.E.J., Jap, T.S., et al. (2007) Subclinical hypothyroidism is a risk factor for nephropathy and cardiovascular diseases in Type 2 diabetic patients. *Diabetic Medicine* 24(12): 1336–1344.

Chen, Y.J., Wu, C.Y., Shen, J.L., et al. (2008) Psoriasis independently associated with hyperleptinemia contributing to metabolic syndrome. *Archive of Dermatology* 144: 1571–1575.

Chew, B-H., Shariff-Ghazali, S., Fernandez, A. (2014) Psychological aspects of diabetes care: effecting behavioural change in patients. *Diabetes Care* 5(6): 796–808.

Chiba, M., Suzuki, S., Hinokio, Y., et al. (2000) Tyrosine hydroxylase gene microsatellite polymorphism associated with insulin resistance in depressive disorder. *Metabolism* 49:1145–1149.

Ch'ng, C.L., Jones, M.K., Kingham, J.G.C. (2007) Celiac disease and autoimmune thyroid disease. *Clinical Medicine and Research* 5(3): 184–192.

Ch'ng, C.L., Biswas, M., Benton, A., et al. (2005) Prospective screening for coeliac disease in patients with Graves' hyperthyroidism using antigliadin and tissue transglutaminase antibodies. *Clinical Endocrinology* 62(3): 303–306.

Ciechanowski, P.S., Katon, W.J., Russo, J.E., et al. (2003) The relationship of depressive symptoms to symptom reporting, self-care, and glucose control in diabetes. *General Hospital Psychiatry* 25: 246–252.

Ciechanowski, P.S., Katon, W.J., Russo, J.E., et al. (2001) The patient-provider relationship: attachment theory and adherence to treatment in diabetes. *General Hospital Psychiatry* 158(1): 29–35.

Ciechanowski, P.S., Katon, W.J., Russo, J.E. (2000) Depression and diabetes: impact of depressive symptoms on adherence, function, and costs. *Archive of Internal Medicine* 160: 3278–3285.

Clark, C.F., Piesowicz, A.T., Spathis, G.S. (1990) Limited joint mobility in children and adolescents with Type 1 diabetes mellitus. *Annals of Rheumatic Disease* 49(4): 236–237.

Clark, M.L. & Utz, S.W. (2014) Social determinants of type 2 diabetes and health in the United States. *World Journal of Diabetes* 5: 296–304.

Clark, M. (2004a) *Understanding Diabetes.* West Sussex, England: John Wiley & Sons Ltd.

Clark, M. (2004b) Identification and treatment of depression in people with diabetes. *Diabetes and Primary Care* 5(3): 124–127.

Coates, P.S., Fernstrom, J.D., Fernstrom, M.H., et al. (2004) Gastric bypass surgery for morbid obesity leads to an increase in bone turnover and a decrease in bone mass. *Journal of Clinical Endocrinology and Metabolism* 89: 1061–1065.

Cohen, A.D., Gilutz, H., Henkin, Y., et al. (2007) Psoriasis and the metabolic syndrome. *Acta Dermatology and Venereology* 87: 506–509.

Cohen, S.T., Welch, G., Jacobson, A.M., et al. (1997) The association of lifetime psychiatric illness and increased retinopathy in patients with type I diabetes mellitus. *Psychosomatics* 38(2):98–108.

Coimbra, S., Oliveira, H., Reis, F., et al. (2010) Circulating adipokine levels in Portuguese patients with psoriasis vulgaris according to body mass index, severity and therapy. *Journal of European Academic Dermatology and Venereology* 24: 1386–1394.

Coiro, V., Volpi, R., Marchesi, C., et al. (1997) Influence of residual C-peptide secretion on nocturnal serum TSH peak in well-controlled diabetic patients. *Clinical Endocrinology* 47(3): 305–310.

Collin, P., Reunala, T., Pukkala, E., et al. (1994) Coeliac disease-associated disorders and survival. *Gut* 35(9): 1215–1218.

Colton, P.A., Rodin, G.M., Olmsted, M.P., et al. (1999) Eating disturbances in young women with Type 1 diabetes mellitus: mechanism and consequences. *Psychiatric Annuls* 29: 213–218.

Colton, P.A., Olmsted, M.P., Daneman, D., et al. (2007) Five-year prevalence & persistence of disturbed eating behaviour and eating disorders in girls with Type 1 diabetes. *Diabetes Care* 30: 2861–2862.

Colton, P.A., Olmsted, M.P., Daneman, D., et al. (2004) Disturbed eating disorders in pre-teen & early teenage girls with Type 1 diabetes: a case-controlled study. *Diabetes Care* 27: 1654–1659.

Connor, M. & Norman, P. (1996) *Predicting Health Behaviour.* Buckingham: Open University Press.

Corrigan, P.W. & McCracken, S.G. (1995a) Refocusing the training of psychiatric rehabilitation staff. *Psychiatric Services* 46(11): 1172–1177.

Corrigan, P.W. & McCracken, S.G. (1995b) Psychiatric rehabilitation and staff development: educational and organizational models. *Clinical Psychology Review* 15: 699–719.

Cosnes, J., Cellier, C., Viola, S., et al. (2008) Incidence of autoimmune diseases in celiac disease: protective effect of the gluten-free diet. *Clinical Gastroenterology and Hepatology* 6 (7): 753–758.

Cox, D., Irvine, A., Gouder-Frederick, L., et al. (1987) Fear of hypoglycaemia: Quantification, validation and utilization. *Diabetes Care* 10(5): 617–621.

Cox, N.H., Gordon, P.M., Dodd, H. (2002) Generalized pustule aranderythrodermic psoriasis associated with bupropion treatment. *British Journal of Dermatology* 146:1061–1063.

Coyne, J.C. (1994) Self-reported distress: analog or Ersatz depression? *Psychology Bulletin* 116: 29–45.

Cranston, I. (2005) *Diabetes and the Brain.* In: Diabetes: Chronic Complications, Shaw, K.M. & Cummings, M.H. (Eds.), second edition. Chichester, West Sussex: John Wiley & Sons Limited.

Criego, A. & Jahraus, J. (2009) Eating disorders and diabetes. *Diabetes Spectrum* 22(3): 143–146.

Criego, A., Scott, M.S., Crow, M.D., et al. (2009) Eating Disorders and Diabetes: Screening and Detection. *Diabetes Spectrum* 22(3): 143–146.

Crookes, P.F. (2006) Surgical treatment of morbid obesity. *Annual Review of Medicine* 57: 243–264.

Crow, S.J., Keel, P.K., Kendall, D. (2000) Relationship of weight and eating disorders in Type 2 diabetic patients: A multicentre study. *International Journal of Eating Disorders* 28: 68-77.

Crow, S.J., Keel, P.K., Kendall, D. (1998) Eating disorders and insulin-dependent diabetes mellitus. *Psychosomatics* 39:233–243.

Cuijpers, P. & Smit, F. (2002) Excess mortality in depression: a meta-analysis of community studies. *Journal of Affective Disorders* 72: 227–236.

Dalle-Grave, R., Calugi, S., Marchesini, G. (2008) Is amenorrhea a useful criterion for the diagnosis of anorexia nervosa? *Behaviour Research Therapy* 46: 1290–1296.

Dalsgaard, E.M., Vestergaard, M., Skriver, M.V., et al. (2014) Psychological distress, cardiovascular complications and mortality among people with screen-detected type 2 diabetes: follow-up of the AD-DITION-Denmark trial. *Diabetologia* 57: 710–717.

Daily Telegraph (2015a) Diabetes 'threat' to NHS' as number of patients passes 3m. *Daily Telegraph*, 17th August 2015.

Daily Telegraph (2015b) Diabetes cases rise by 65pc in 10 years. *Daily Telegraph*, 15th October 2015.

Daneman, D., Rodin, G., Jones, J., et al. (2002) Eating disorders in adolescent girls and young women with Type 1 diabetes. *Diabetes Spectrum* 15(2): 83–105.

Dandona, P., Fonesca, V., Meir, A., et al. (1983) Diarrhea and Metformin in a diabetes clinic. *Diabetes Care* 6(5): 472–474.

Dantzer, R. (2004) Cytokine-induced sickness behaviour: a neuroimmune response to activation of innate immunity. *European Journal of Pharmacology* 500: 399–411.

Dantzer, R. (2001) Cytokine-induced sickness behavior: where do we stand? *Brain Behaviour and Immunity* 15: 7–24.

Danzer, G., Mulzer, J., Weber, G., et al. (2005) Advanced anorexia nervosa, associated with pneumomediastinum, pneumothorax, and soft-tissue emphysema without esophageal lesion. *International Journal of Eating Disorders* 38: 281–284.

Davidson, K., Jonahs, B.S., Dixon, K.E., et al. (2000) Do depression symptoms predict early hypertension incidence in young adults in the CARDIA study? Coronary Artery Risk Development in Young Adults. *Archive of Internal Medicine* 160(10): 1495–1500.

Davis, E.A., Soong, S.A., Byrne, G.C., et al. (1996) Acute hyperglycemia impairs cognitive function in children with IDDM. *Journal of Pediatric Endocrinology and Metabolism* 9: 455–461.

Das-Munshi, J., Stewart, R., Ismail, K., et al. (2007) Diabetes, common mental disorders, and disability: findings from the UK National Psychiatric Morbidity Survey. *Psychosomatic Medicine* 69: 543–550.

Day, J.L. (1995) Why should patients do what we ask them to do? *Patient Education and Counselling* 26 (1–3): 113-118.

De Caprio, C., Alfano, A., Senatore, I. (2006) Severe acute liver damage in anorexia nervosa: two case reports. *Nutrition* 22: 572–575.

Deci, E.L. & Ryan, R.M. (2000) The "What" and "Why" of goal pursuits: human needs and the self determination of behaviour. *Psychological Inquiry*, 11(4): 227–268.

De Groot, M., Anderson, R., Freedland, K.E., et al. (2001) Association of depression and diabetes complications: a meta-analysis. *Psychosomatic Medicine* 63: 619–630.

Den Hollander, J.G., Wulkan, R.W., Mantel, M.J., et al. (2005) Correlation between severity of thyroid dysfunction and renal function. *Clinical Endocrinology* 62(4): 423–427.

Department of Health (2005) *Structured Patient Education in Diabetes: Report from the Patient Education Working Group.* Department of Health: London, England.
http:// www.diabetes.org.uk/Documents/Reports/ StructuredPatientEd.pdf

Department of Health (2003a) *National Service Framework for Diabetes: Standards Document.* London: Department of Health.

Department of Health (2003b) *National Service Framework for Diabetes.* London: Department of Health.

Department of Health (2002) *Priorities for the Diabetes National Service Framework (NSF) for England and Wales.* www.doh.gov.uk/nsf/diabetes

Department of Health (2001) *National Service Framework for Diabetes.* Bit.ly/DHNSFDiabetes

De Rubeis, R.J., Evans, M.D., Hollon, S.D., et al. (1990) How does cognitive therapy work? Cognitive change and symptom change in cognitive therapy and pharmacotherapy for depression. *Journal of Consulting Clinical Psychology* 58(6): 862–869.

Dew, M.A. (1998) *Psychiatric Disorder in the Context of Physical Illness. Adversity, Stress, and Psychopathology.* New York: Oxford University Press.

de Zwaan, M., Hilbert, A., Swan-Kremeier, L., et al. (2010) Comprehensive interview assessment of eating behavior 18-35 months after gastric bypass surgery for morbid obesity. *Surgery for Obesity and Related Diseases* 6(1): 79–85.

Diabetes Control and Complications Trial Research Group (1993) The effect of intensified treatment on the development and progression of long-term complications of insulin dependent diabetes mellitus. *New England Journal of Medicine* 329: 977–986.

Diabetes UK (17th August 2015) 10% of the NHS budget is spent on treating diabetes. www.diabetes.co.uk

Diabetes UK (2012) Diabetes in the UK 2010: Key statistics on diabetes. London: Diabetes UK. Bit.ly/DiabetesUKStats2010

Diabetes UK (2008) *Early Identification of Type 2 Diabetes and the new Vascular Risk Assessment and Management Programme.* Position Statement Update. London: Diabetes UK.

Diabetes UK (2006) *Diabetes Information Jigsaw Report.* London: Diabetes UK.

Diabetes UK (2000) *What Diabetes Care to Expect.* London: Diabetes UK.

Diamanti, A., Ferretti, F., Guglielmi, R., et al. (2011) Thyroid autoimmunity in children with coeliac disease: a prospective survey. *Archives of Disease in Childhood* 96(11): 1038–1041.

Dimitriadis, G., Mitrou, P., Lambadiari, V., et al. (2006) Insulin action in adipose tissue and muscle in hypothyroidism. *Journal of Clinical Endocrinology and Metabolism* 91(12): 4930–4937.

Dimitriadis, G., Parry-Billings, M., Bevan, S., et al. (1997) The effects of insulin on transport and metabolism of glucose in skeletal muscle from hyperthyroid and hypothyroid rats. *European Journal of Clinical Investigation* 27(6): 475–483.

Dimitriadis, G., Baker, B., Marsh, H. (1985) Effect of thyroid hormone excess on action, secretion, and metabolism of insulin in humans. *The American Journal of Physiology* 248(5): E593–E601.

DiMatteo, M.R., Lepper, H.S., Croghan, T.W. (2000) Depression is a risk factor for noncompliance with medical treatment: meta-analysis of the effects of anxiety and depression on patient adherence. *Archive of Internal Medicine* 160: 2101–2107.

Dishman, R.K. (1986) Exercise compliance: a new view for public health. *Physician and Sports Medicine*14: 127–145.

Dixon, A. (2008) *Motivation and Confidence: What Does it Take to Change Behaviour?* The Kings Fund: London, England.

Dixon, J.B., O'Brien, P.E., Playfair, J., et al. (2008) Laparoscopic adjustable gastric banding in severely obese adolescents: a randomized trial. *Journal of the American Medical Association* 299: 316–323.

Docx, M.K., Gewillig, M., Simons, A., et al. (2010) Pericardial effusions in adolescent girls with anorexia nervosa: clinical course and risk factors. *Eating Disorde*rs 18: 218–225.

Douek, I.F., Leech, N.J., Gillmor, H.A., et al. (1999) Children with type 1 diabetes and their unaffected siblings have fewer symptoms of asthma. *Lancet* 353:1850.

Domargard, A., Sarnbad, S., Kroon, M., et al. (1999) Increased prevalence of overweight in adolescent girls with type 1 diabetes mellitus. *Pediatrics* 88: 1223–1228.

Donkin, L., Ellis, C.J., Powell, R., et al. (2006) Illness perceptions predict reassurance following a negative exercise stress testing result. *Psychology and Health* 21: 421–430.

Donnovan, P.T., MacDonald, T.M., Morris, A.D. (2002) Adherence to prescribed oral hypoglycaemic medications in a population of patients with type 2 diabetes: a retrospective cohort study. *Diabetic Medicine* 19: 274–284.

Draelos, M.T., Jacobson, A.M., Weinger, K., et al. (1995) Cognitive function in patients with insulin-dependent diabetes mellitus during hyperglycemia and hypoglycemia. *American Journal of Medicine* 98: 135–144.

Drucker, D.J., Sherman, S.I., Gorelick, F.S. (2010) Incretin-based therapies for the treatment of type 2 diabetes: evaluation of the risks and benefits. *Diabetes Care* 33: 428– 433.

Druss, B.G., Rohrbaugh, R.M., Rosenheck, R.A. (2000) Depressive symptoms and health costs in older medical patients. *General Hospital Psychiatry* 156(3):477–479.

Duckworth, A.L. (2011) The significance of self-control. *Proceedings of the National Academy of Science* 108: 2639–2640.

Dymek, M.P., le Grange, D., Neven, K., et al. (2001) Quality of life and psychosocial adjustment in patients after Roux-en-Y gastric Bypass: a brief report. *Obesity Surgery* 11(1): 32–39.

Eaton, W.W., Armenian, H., Gallo, J., et al. (1996) Depression and the risk for onset of type II diabetes. *Diabetes Care* 19: 1097–1102.

Eckel, R., Grundy, S., Zimmet, P. (2005) The metabolic syndrome. *Lancet* 365: 1415–1428.

Eder, K., Baffy, N., Falus, A., Fulop, A.K. (2009) The major inflammatory mediator interleukin-6 and obesity. *Inflammation. Research* 58: 727–736.

Egede, L.E., Zheng, D., Simpson, K. (2002) Comorbid depression is associated with increased health care use and expenditures in individuals with diabetes. *Diabetes Care* 25(3): 464-470.

Ehrlich, S., Burghardt, R., Weiss, D., et al. (2008) Glial and neuronal damage markers in patients with anorexia nervosa. *Journal of Neurological Transmission* 115: 921–927.

Eisenberg, N. (2000) Emotion, Regulation, and Moral Development. *Annual Review of Sociology* 51: 665–697.

Elfstrom, P., Montgomery, S.M., Kampe, O., et al. (2008) Risk of thyroid disease in individuals with celiac disease. *The Journal of Clinical Endocrinology and Metabolism* 93(10): 3915–3921.

Elfstrom, P., Montgomery, S.M., Kampe, O., et al. (2007) Risk of primary adrenal insufficiency in patients with celiac disease. *The Journal of Clinical Endocrinology and Metabolism* 92(9): 3595–3598.

Emanuele, N.V., Swade, T.F., Emanuele, M.A. (1998) Consequences of alcohol use in diabetics. *Alcohol Health & Research World* 22(3): 211–219.

Engström, I., Kroon, M., Arvidsson, C.G., et al. (1997) Subclinical and clinical eating disorders in IDDM negatively affect metabolic control. *Diabetes Care* 20: 182–184.

Erdogan, M., Canataraglu, A., Ganidaqil, S., et al. (2011) Metabolic syndrome prevalence in subclinic and overt hypothyroid patients and the relation among metabolic syndrome parameters. *Journal of Endocrinological Investigation* 34(7): 488–492.

Erickson, S.J., Robinson, T.N., Farish-Haydel, K., et al. (2000) Are overweight children unhappy? Body mass index, depressive symptoms, and overweight concerns in elementary school children. *Archives of Pediatrics & Adolescent Medicine* 154(9): 931–935.

Estour, B., Germain, .N., Diconne, E. (2010) Hormonal profile heterogeneity and short-term physical risk in restrictive anorexia nervosa. *Journal of Clinical Endocrinology and Metabolism.* 95: 2203–2210.

Ettigi, P. & Brown, G. (1977) Psychoneuroendocrinology of affective disorder: an overview. *American Journal of Psychiatry* 134: 493–501.

Fairburn, C.G., Peveler, R.C., Davis, B., et al. (1991) Eating disorders with young adults with insulin dependent diabetes mellitus: a controlled study. *British Medical Journal* 303: 17–20.

Farmer, M.E., Locke, B.Z., Moscicki, E.K., et al. (1988) Physical activity and depressive symptoms: the NHANES I Epidemiologic Follow-up Study. *American Journal of Epidemiology* 128(6): 1340–1351.

Fasino, A., Berti, I., Gerarduzzi, T., et al. (2003) Prevalence of celiac disease in at-risk and not-at-risk groups in the United States: a large multicenter study. *Archives of Internal Medicine* 163 (3): 286–292.

Fava, G.A., Grandi, S., Zielezny, M., et al. (1996) Four-year outcome for cognitive behavioral treatment of residual symptoms in major depression. *General Hospital Psychiatry* 153(7): 945–947.

Fazeli, P.K. & Klibanski, A. (2014) Bone metabolism in anorexia nervosa. *Current Osteoporosis Report* 12: 82–89.

Fechner-Bates, S., Coyne, J.C., Schwenk, T.L. (1994) The relationship of self-reported distress to depressive disorders and other psychopathology. *Journal of Consulting Clinical Psychology* 62: 550–559.

Felig, P. (1979) Starvation. In: *Endocrinology.* DeGroot, L.J. (Ed.) New York: Grune & Stratton.

Fernandez, A.Z. Jr., DeMaria, E.J., Tichansky, D.S., et al. (2004) Experience with over 3,000 open and laparoscopic bariatric procedures: multivariate analysis of factors related to leak and resultant mortality. *Surgery and Endoscopy* 18: 193–197.

Fiorentino, T.V., Prioletta, A., Zuo, P., et al. (2013) Hyperglycemia-induced oxidative stress and its role in diabetes mellitus related cardiovascular diseases. *Current Pharmaceutical Design* 19: 5695–5703.

Fisher, L., Gonzalez, J.S., Polonsky, W.H. (2014) The confusing tale of depression and distress in patients with diabetes: a call for greater clarity and precision. *Diabetes Medicine* 31: 764–772.

Fisher, L., Mullan, J.T., Arean, P., et al. (2010) Diabetes distress but not clinical depression or depressive symptoms is associated with glycemic control in both cross-sectional and longitudinal analyses. *Diabetes Care* 33: 23–28.

Fisher, L. & Ransom, D.C. (1997) Developing a strategy for managing behavioral health care within the context of primary care. *Archive of Family Medi*cine 6(4): 324–333.

Fitzgerald, R., Saddler, M., Connolly, M., et al. (2014) Psoriasis and insulin resistance: a review. *Journal of Diabetes Research and Clinical Metabolism* http://www/hoajonline.com/journals/pdf2050-0866-3-3.pdf

Folkman, S. & Moskowitz, J.T. (2000) Positive affect and the other side of coping. *American Psychology* 55: 647–654.

Forjuoh, S.N., Ory, M.G., Jiang, L., et al. (2014) Impact of chronic disease self-management programs on type 2 diabetes management in primary care. *World Journal of Diabetes* 5: 407–414.

Fortune, D.G., Richards, H.L., Kirby, B., et al. (2003) Psychological distress impairs clearance of psoriasis in patients treated with photochemotherapy. *Archive of Dermatology* 139:752–756.

Fortune, D.G., Richards, H.L., Main, C.J., et al. (2000) Pathological worrying, illness perceptions and disease severity in patients with psoriasis. *British Journal of Health Psychology* 5: 71–82.

Fortune, D.G., Richards, H.L., Main, C.J., et al. (1998) What patients with psoriasis believe about their condition. *Journal of the American Academy of Dermatology* 39: 196–201.

Fowler, M.J. (2008) Microvascular and Macrovascular Complications of Diabetes. *Clinical Diabetes* 26: 77–82.

Frasure-Smith, N., Lesperance, F., Talajic, M. (1993) Depression following myocardial infarction. Impact on 6-month survival. *Journal of the American Medical Association* 270(15): 1819–1825.

Freedland, K.E. (2004) Section II: Hypothesis 1: Depression is a risk factor for the development of type 2 diabetes. *Diabetes Spectrum* 17: 150–152.

Fredrickson, L. (Ed.) (1995) *The Insulin Pump Therapy Book.* Los Angeles, California: MiniMed Technologies.

French, S.A., Story, M., Perry, C.L. (1995) Self-esteem and obesity in children and adolescents: a literature review. *Obesity Research* 3(5): 479–490.

Friedman, M.A. & Brownell, K.D. (1995) Psychological correlates of obesity: moving to the next research generation. *Psychological Bulletin* 117(1): 3–20.

Frigg, A., Peterli, R., Peters, T., et al. (2004) Reduction in co-morbidities 4 years after laparoscopic adjustable gastric banding. *Obesity Surgery* 14(2): 216–223.

Gale, L., Vedhara, K., Searle, A., et al. (2008) Patients' perspectives on foot complication in Type 2 diabetes: A qualitative study. *British Journal of General Practice*. doi: 10:3399/bjgp08X31957.

Gavard, J.A., Lustman, P.J., Clouse, R.E. (1993) Prevalence of depression in adults with diabetes: an epidemiological evaluation. *Diabetes Care* 16: 1167–1178.

Gary, T.L., Crum, R.M., Cooper-Patrick, L., et al. (2000) Depressive symptoms and metabolic control in African-Americans with type 2 diabetes. *Diabetes Care* 23(1): 23–29.

Gask, L., Macdonald, W., Bower, P. (2011) What is the relationship between diabetes and depression? A qualitative meta-synthesis of patient experience of co-morbidity. *Chronic Illness* 7: 239–252.

Gaudiani, J.L., Sabel, A.L., Mascolo, M. (2012) Severe anorexia nervosa: outcomes from a medical stabilization unit. *International Journal of Eating Disorders* 45: 85–92.

Gervey, B., Igou, E., Trope, Y. (2005) Positive mood and future-oriented self-evaluation. *Motivation and Emotion* 29: 267–294.

Ghiadoni, L., Donald, A.E., Cropley, M., et al. (2000) Mental stress induces transient endothelial dysfunction in humans. *Circulation* 102: 2473–2478.

Giacco, F. & Brownlee, M. (2010) Oxidative stress and diabetic complications. *Circulation Research* 107: 1058–1070.

Gill, D. & Hatcher, S. (2000) Antidepressants for depression in medical illness [update software]. *Cochrane Database Systematic Review* (4): CD 001312.

Given, C.W., Given, B.A., Galin, R.S., et al. (1983) Development of scales to measure beliefs of diabetes patients. *Research in Nursing and Health* 6: 127–141.

Glasgow, R.E., Fisher, E.B., Anderson, B.J. (1999) Behavioural science in diabetes. *Diabetes Care* 22(5): 21–29.

Gobel-Fabbri, A.E., Fifkan, J., Franco, D., et al. (2008) Insulin restriction and associated morbidity and mortality in women with type 1 diabetes. *Diabetes Care* 31(3): 415–419.

Golden, S.H., Lazo, M., Carnethon, M., et al. (2008) Examining a bidirectional association between depressive symptoms and diabetes. *Journal of the American Medical Association* 299: 2751–2759.

Goldney, R.D., Phillips, P.J., Fisher, L.J. (2004) Diabetes, depression, and quality of life: a population study. *Diabetes Care* 27: 1066–1070.

Golin, C.E., DiMatteo, M.R., Gelberg, L. (2001) The role of participation in the doctor-patient visit. *Diabetes Care* 19: 1153–1164.

Goodman, E. & Whitaker, R.C. (2002) A prospective study of the role of depression in the development and persistence of adolescent obesity. *Pediatrics* 110(3): 497–504.

Gordon, K.B., Langley, R.G., Lenardi, C., et al. (2006) Clinical response to adalimumab treatment in patients with moderate to severe psoriasis: double-blind, randomized controlled trial and open-label extension study. *Journal of the American Academy of Dermatology* 55: 598–606.

Gray, J.R. & Bias, A. (1999) Toward short-term thinking in threat-related negative emotional states. *Proceedings of the Social Psychology Bureau* 25: 65–75.

Greco, D., Pisciotta, M., Gambina, F., et al. (2013) Celiac disease in subjects with type 1 diabetes mellitus: a prevalence study in western Sicily (Italy). *Endocrine* 43(1): 108– 111.

Gross, J.J. (2003) Emotion regulation: affective, cognitive, and social consequences. *Psychophysiology* 39: 281–291.

Gschwend, S., Ryan, C., Atchison, J., et al. (1995) Effects of acute hyperglycemia on mental efficiency and counter-regulatory hormones in adolescents with insulin-dependent diabetes mellitus. *Journal of Pediatrics* 126: 178–184.

Guisado, J.A., Vaz, J.F., Alarcon, J., et al. (2002) Psychopathological status and interpersonal functioning following weight loss in morbidly obese patients undergoing bariatric surgery. *Obesity Surgery* 12(6): 835–840.

Gupta, M.A., Schork, N.J., Gupta, A.K., et al. (1993) Suicidal ideation in psoriasis. *International Journal of Dermatology* 32: 188–90.

Gupta, M.A., Gupta, A.K., Kirkby, S., et al. (1989) Apsychocutaneous profile or psoriasis patients who are stress reactors: a study of 127 patients. General Hospital Psychiatry 11: 166–173.

Guo, J.J., Keck, P.E. Jr., Corey-Lisle, P.K., et al. (2007) Risk of diabetes mellitus associated with atypical antipsychotic use among Medicaid patients with bipolar disorder: A nested case-control study. *Pharmacotherapy* 27: 27–35.

Hadithi, M., de Boer, H., Meijer, J.W.R., et al. (2007) Coeliac disease in Dutch patients with Hashimoto's thyroiditis and vice versa. *World Journal of Gastroenterology* 13(11): 1715–1722.

Hagander, B., Berg, N.O., Brandt, L., et al. (1977) Hepatic injury in adult coeliac disease. *Lancet* 2 (8032): 270–272.

Hage, M., Zantout, M.S., Azar, S.I. (2011) Thyroid disorders and diabetes mellitus. *Journal of Thyroid Research* doi: 10: 4061/2011/439463.

Hagger, M.S. (2013) The multiple pathways by which self-control predicts behavior. *Frontiers of Psychology* 4: 849.

Hall, R., Joseph, D.H., Schwartz-Barcott, E.L. (2003) Overcoming obstacles to behavioural change in diabetes self-management. *The Diabetes Educator* 292(2): 303–311.

Hammes, H.P. (2003) Pathophysiological mechanisms of diabetic angiopathy. *Journal of Diabetes Complications* 17: 16–19.

Hanninen, J.A., Takala, J.K., Keinanen-Kiukaanniemi, S.M. (1999) Depression in subjects with type 2 diabetes. Predictive factors and relation to quality of life. *Diabetes Care* 22(6): 997–998.

Harder, H., Dinesen, B., Astrup, A. (2004) The effect of rapid weight loss on lipid profile and glycaemic control in obese Type 2 diabetic patients. *International Journal of Obesity* 28: 180–182.

Harris, R.H., Sasson, G., Mehler, P.S. (2013) Elevation of liver function tests in severe anorexia nervosa. *International Journal of Eating Disorders* 46: 369–374.

Hassmen, P., Koivula, N., Uutela, A. (2000) Physical exercise and psychological well-being: a population study in Finland. *Preventative Medicine* 30(1): 17–25.

Haviland, M.G., Dial, T.H., McGhee, W.H., et al. (2001) Depression and satisfaction with health plans. *Psychiatric Services* 52(3): 279.

Heather, N. & Robertson, I. (1997) *Problem Drinking.* Oxford: Oxford University Press.

Hemlock, C., Rosenthal, J.S., Winston, A. (1992) Fluoxetine-induced psoriasis. *Annals of Pharmacotherapy* 26: 211–212.

Hermanns, N., Caputo, S., Dzida, G., et al. (2013) Screening, evaluation and management of depression in people with diabetes in primary care. *Primary Care Diabetes* 7: 1-10.

Herpertz, S., Kielmann, R., Wolf, A.M., et al. (2003) Does obesity surgery improve psychosocial functioning? A systematic review. *International Journal of Obesity* 27(11): 1300–1314.

Herpertz, S., Albus, C., Kielmann, R., et al. (2001) Comorbidity of diabetes mellitus and eating disorders: a follow-up study. *Journal of Psychosomatic Research* 51: 673–678.

Herpertz, S., Albus, C., Kielmann, R., et al. (1998) Eating disorders and insulin-dependent diabetes mellitus. *Psychosomatics* 39: 233–243.

Herzog, W., Deter, H.C., Fiehn, W., et al. (1997) Medical findings and predictors of long-term physical outcome in anorexia nervosa: a prospective, 12-year follow-up study. *Psychology Medicine.* 27: 269–279.

Hettema, J., Steele, J., Miller, W.R. (2005) Motivational interviewing. *Annual Review of Clinical Psychology* 1: 91–111.

Herrin, M. (2003) *Nutrition Counseling in the Treatment of Eating Disorders.* New York: Brunner-Routledge 3: 27–39.

Heneghan, M.A., Mchugh, P., Stevens, F.M., et al. (1997) Addison's disease and selective IgA deficiency in two coeliac patients. *Scandinavian Journal of Gastroenterology* 32(5): 509–511.

Higgs, M.L., Wade, T., Cescato, M., et al. (1997) Differences between treatment seekers in an obese population: medical intervention vs. dietary restriction. *Journal of Behavioral Medicine* 20(4): 391–406.

Himmerich, H., Fulda, S., Linseisen, J., et al. (2008) Depression, comorbidities and the TNF-alpha system. *European Psychiatry* 23: 421–429.

Hirakawa, Y., Arima, H., Zoungas, S., et al. (2014) Impact of visit-to-visit glycemic variability on the risks of macrovascular and microvascular events and all-cause mortality in type 2 diabetes: the ADVANCE trial. *Diabetes Care* 37: 2359–2365.

Hirshberg, B., Muszkat, M., Marom, T., et al. (2000) Natural course of insulin edema. *Journal of Endocrinology Investigation* 23(3): 187–188.

Ho, N., Sommers, M.S., Lucki, I. (2013) Effects of diabetes on hippocampal neurogenesis: links to cognition and depression. *Neuroscience and Biobehavior Review* 37: 1346–1362.

Hochlehnert, A., Löwe, B., Bludau, H.B., et al. (2010) Spontaneous pneumomediastinum in anorexia nervosa: a case report and review of the literature on pneumomediastinum and pneumothorax. *European Eating Disorders Review* 18: 107–115.

Hoffman, R.G., Speelman, D.J., Hinnen, D.A., et al. (1989) Changes in cortical functioning with acute hypoglycemia and hyperglycemia in type 1 diabetes. *Diabetes Care* 12:193–197.

Hogan, A.E., Tobin, A.M., Ahern, T., et al. (2011) Glucagon-like peptide-1 (GLP-1) and the regulation of human invariant natural killer T cells: lessons from obesity, diabetes and psoriasis. *Diabetologia* 54: 2745–2754.

Höke, U., Thijssen, J., Bommel, R van V., et al. (2013) Influence of diabetes on left ventricular systolic and diastolic function and on long-term outcome after cardiac resynchronization therapy. *Diabetes Care* 36(4): 985–991.

Holford, P. (2011) *Say No to Diabetes: 10 Secrets to Preventing and Reversing Diabetes.* London: Little Brown (Piatkus).

Holmes, C.S., Hayford, J.T., Gonzalez, J.L., et al. (1983) A survey of cognitive functioning at different glucose levels in diabetic persons. *Diabetes Care* 6: 180–185.

Holmes, S.R., Gudridge, T.A., Gaudiani, J.L. (2012) Dysphagia in severe anorexia nervosa and potential therapeutic intervention: a case series. *Annuls of Otology, Rhinology and Laryngology* 121: 449–456.

Holt, R.I., de Groot, M., Lucki, I., et al. (2014) NIDDK international conference report on diabetes and depression: current understanding and future directions. *Diabetes Care* 37: 2067–2077.

Holt, R.I., Nicolucci, A., Burns, K., et al. (2013) Diabetes Attitudes, Wishes and Needs second study (DAWNN): cross-national comparisons on barriers and resources for optimal care--healthcare professional perspective. *Diabetes Medicine* 30: 789–798.

Holton, S.D., DeRubeis, S., Evans, M.D., et al. (1992) Cognitive therapy and pharmacotherapy for depression singly and in combination. *Archives of General Psychiatry* 49: 774–781.

Horne, R. (1997) Representation of medicine and treatment: advances in theory and measurement. In: Petrie, K.J., Weinmann, J. (Eds.) *Perceptions of Health and Illness: Current Research and Applications.* London: Harwood Academic, 155–188.

Hsia, Y-T., Cheng, W-C., Liao, W-C., et al. (2015) Type 1 diabetes and increased risk of subsequent asthma: a nationwide population-based cohort study. *Medicine* 94(36): pe1466.

Hsia, D.S., Fallon, S.C., Brandt, M.L. (2012) Adolescent Bariatric Surgery. *Archives of Pediatric & Adolescent Medicine* 166(8): 757–766.

Hsu, Y.Y., Chen, B.H., Huang, M.C., et al. (2009) Disturbed eating behaviour in Taiwanese adolescents with Type 1 diabetes mellitus: A comparative study. *Pediatric Diabetes* 10: 74–81.

Hylan, T., Crown, W.H., Meneades, L., et al. (1999) SSRI antidepressant drug use patterns in the naturalistic setting: a multivariate analysis. *Medical Care* 37 (4 Lilly supplement): AS36–AS44.

Hu, T., Zhang, D., Wang, J., et al. (2014) Relation between emotion regulation and mental health: a meta-analysis review. *Psychological Report* 114: 341–362.

Illman, J., Corringham, R., Robinson, D. Jr., et al. (2005) Areinflammatory cytokines the common link between cancer-associated cachexia and depression? *Journal of Support Oncology* 3: 37–50.

Ikeda, R.M., Kresnow, M.J., Mercy, J.A., et al. (2001) Medical conditions and nearly lethal suicide attempts. *Suicide and Life Threatening Behaviour* 32: 60–67.

Inagaki, T., Yamamoto, M., Tsubouchi, K., et al. (2003) Echocardiographic investigation of pericardial effusion in a case of anorexia nervosa. *International Journal of Eating Disorders* 33: 364–366.

Irvine, W.J. & Barnes, E.W. (1972) Adrenal insufficiency. *Clinical Endocrinology and Metabolism* 1: 549–594.

Ismail, K., Winkley, K., Stahl, D., et al. (2007) A cohort study of people with diabetes and their first foot ulcer: the role of depression on mortality. *Diabetes Care* 30(6):1473–1479.

Izard, C.E. (2009) Emotion theory and research: highlights, unanswered questions, and emerging issues. *Annual Review of Psychology* 60: 1–25.

Izard, C.E. (2007) Basic emotions, natural kinds, emotion schemas, and a new paradigm. *Perspectives on Psychological Science* 2: 260–280.

Jackson, J.L. & Kroenke, K. (1999) Difficult patient encounters in the ambulatory clinic: clinical predictors and outcomes. *Archive of Internal Medicine* 159(10): 1069–1075.

Jacob, S. & Serrano-Gil, M. (2010) Engaging and empowering patients to manage their type 2 diabetes, Part II: Initiatives for success. *Advanced Therapy* 27: 665–680.

Jacobson, A.M., De Groot, M., Samson, J.A. (1997) The effects of psychiatric disorders and symptoms on quality of life in patients with type I and type II diabetes mellitus. *Quality of Life Research* 6(1):11-20.

Jacobson, L. & Sapolsky, R. (1991) The role of the hippocampus in feedback regulation of the hypothalamic-pituitary-adrenocortical axis. *Endocrinology Review* 12: 118–134.

Janis, T. & Mann, L. (1977) *Decision Making: A Psychological Analysis of Conflict, Choice and Commitment.* New York: Collier McMillan.

Janz, N.K. & Becker, M.H. (1984) The Health Belief Model: A decade later. *Health Education Quarterly* 11: 147.

Jaremka, L.M., Lindgren, M.E., Kiecolt-Glaser, J.K. (2013) Synergistic relationships among stress, depression, and troubled relationships: insights from psychoneuroimmunology. *Depression and Anxiety* 30: 288–296.

Jarvholm, K., Olbers, T., Marcus, C., et al. (2012) Short-term psychological outcomes in severely obese adolescents after bariatric surgery. *Obesity* 20(2): 318–323.

Jarvis, S. & Rubin, A.L. (2003) *Diabetes For Dummies.* Chichester: John Wiley & Sons Limited.

Jaser, S.S., Patel, N., Rothman, R.L., et al. (2014) Check it! A randomized pilot of a positive psychology intervention to improve adherence in adolescents with type 1 diabetes. *Diabetes Educator* 40: 659–667.

Jeffcoate, W.J. & Harding, K.G. (2003) Diabetic foot ulcers. *Lancet* 361(9368): 1545–1551.

Jehle, P.M., Jehle, D.R., Mohan, S., et al. (1998) Serum levels of insulin-like growth factor system components and relationship to bone metabolism in type I and type 2 diabetes mellitus patients. *Journal of Endocrinology* 159: 297–306.

Jenny, J.L. (1984) A comparison of four age groups' adaption to diabetes. *Canadian Journal of Public Health* 75: 237–244.

Jensen, P., Thyssen, J.P., Zachariae, C., et al. (2013) Cardiovascular risk factors in subjects with psoriasis: a cross-sectional general population study. *International Journal of Dermatology* 52: 681–583.

Johnson, C. (1985) Initial consultation for patients with bulimia and anorexia nervosa. In *Handbook of Psychotherapy for Anorexia Nervosa and Bulimia.* Garner, D.M., Garfinkel, P.E. (Eds.) New York: Guilford Press.

Johnston, A., Arnadottir, S., Gudjonsson, J.E., et al. (2008) Obesity in psoriasis: leptin and resistin as mediators of cutaneous inflammation. *British Journal of Dermatology* 159: 342–350.

Jonas, B.S. & Mussolino, M.E. (2000) Symptoms of depression as a prospective risk factor for stroke. *Psychosomatic Medicine* 62(4): 463–471.

Jones, J.M., Lawson, M.L., Danemam, D., et al. (2000) Eating disorders in adolescent females with and without type 1 diabetes: cross sectional study. *British Medical Journal* 320: 1563–1566.

Kalarchian, M.A., Marcus, M.D., Levine, M.D., et al. (2007) Psychiatric disorders among bariatric surgery candidates: relationship to obesity and functional health status. *American Journal of Psychiatry* 164(2): 328–334.

Kalmann, R. & Mourits, M.P. (1999) Diabetes mellitus: a risk factor for patients with Graves' orbitopathy. *British Journal of Ophthalmology* 83(4): 463–465.

Kamal, N., Chami, T., Andersen, A. (1991) Delayed gastrointestinal transit times in anorexia nervosa and bulimia nervosa. *Gastroenterology* 101:1320–1324.

Kaminsky, J. & Gadaleta, D. (2002) A study of discrimination within the medical community as viewed by obese patients. *Obesity Surgery* 12(1): 14–18.

Kang, S.M. & Shaver, P.R. (2004) Individual differences in emotional complexity: their psychological implications. *Journal of Personality* 72: 687–726.

Kaplan, R.M., Chadwick, M.W., Schimmel, L.E., et al. (1985) Social Learning interventions to promote metabolic control in type 1 diabetes mellitus: pilot experiment results. *Diabetes Care* 8L: 152–155.

Kaplan, R.M., Aitkins, C.J., Reinsch, S. (1984) Specific efficacy expectations mediate exercise compliance in patients with COPD. *Health Psychology* 3: 223–242.

Karlson, B. & Agardh, C.D. (1997) Burden of illness, metabolic control, and complications in relation to depressive symptoms in IDDM patients. *Diabetic Medicine* 14: 1066–1072.

Karlsson, J., Sjostrom, L., Sullivan, M. (1998) Swedish obese subjects (SOS) — an intervention study of obesity. Two-year follow-up of health-related quality of life (HRQL) and eating behavior after gastric surgery for severe obesity. *International Journal of Obesity* 22(2): 113–126.

Karadag, A.S., Yavuz, B., Ertugrul, D.T., et al. (2010) Is psoriasis a pre-atherosclerotic disease? Increased insulin resistance and impaired endothelial function in patients with psoriasis. *International Journal of Dermatology* 49: 642–646.

Kastner, S., Salbach-Andrae, H., Renneberg, B. (2012) Echocardiographic findings in adolescents with anorexia nervosa at beginning of treatment and after weight recovery. *European Child and Adolescent Psychiatry* 21: 15–21.

Katsilambros, N., Kanka-Gantenbein, C., Liatis, S., et al. (2011) *Diabetic Emergencies and Clinical Management.* Chichester, West Sussex: Wiley-Blackwell.

Katon, W.J. (2003) Clinical and health services relationships between major depression, depressive symptoms, and general medical illness. *Biological Psychiatry* 54: 216–226.

Katon, W.J., Lin, E.H., Von Korff, M., et al. (2010) Collaborative care for patients with depression and chronic illnesses. *New England Journal of Medicine* 363: 2611–2620.

Katon, W.J., Von Korff, M., Lin, E., et al. (1995) Collaborative management to achieve treatment guidelines. Impact on depression in primary care. *Journal of the American Medical Association* 273(13):1026–1031.

Katz, J. & Peberdy, A. (2001) *Promoting Health, Knowledge and Practice.* London: Palgrave Macmillan.

Kelly, S.D., Howe, C.J., Hendler, J.P., et al. (2005) Disordered eating behaviors in youth with type 1 diabetes. *Diabetes Educator* 34: 572–583.

Kawamura, T., Shioiri, T., Takahashi, K., et al. (2007) Survival rate and causes of mortality in the elderly with depression: a 15-year prospective study of a Japanese community sample, the Matsunoyama-Niigata suicide prevention project. *Journal of Investigative Medicine* 55: 106–114.

Keidar, A. (2011) Bariatric surgery for Type 2 diabetes reversal: the risks. *Diabetes Care* 34(2): S361–S367.

Keidar, A., Appelbaum, L., Schweiger, C., et al. (2010) Dilated upper sleeve can be associated with severe postoperative gastroesophageal dysmotility and reflux. *Obesity Surgery* 20: 140–147.

Keidar, A., Szold, A., Carmon, E., et al. (2005) Band slippage after laparoscopic adjustable gastric banding: etiology and treatment. *Surgical Endoscopy* 19: 262–267.

Kemp, H.F., Hundal, H.S., Taylor, P.M. (1997) Glucose transport correlates with GLUT2 abundance in rat liver during altered thyroid status. *Molecular and Cellular Endocrinology* 128(1-2): 97–102.

Keshavan, M.S., Vinogradov, S., Rumsey, J., et al. (2014) Cognitive training in mental disorders: update and future directions. *American Journal of Psychiatry* 171: 510–522.

Kessing, L.V., Nilsson, F.M., Siersma, V., et al. (2004) Increased risk of developing diabetes in depressive and bipolar disorders? *Journal of Psychiatric Research* 38: 395–402.

Kessing, L.V., Nilsson, F.M., Siersma, V., et al. (2003) No increased risk of developing depression in diabetes compared to other chronic illness. *Diabetes Research and Clinical Practice* 62 (2): 113–121.

Kiecolt-Glaser, J.K., McGuire, L., Robles, T.F., et al. (2002a) Emotions, morbidity, and mortality: new perspectives from psychoneuroimmunology. *Annual Review of Psychology* 53: 83–107.

Kiecolt-Glaser, J.K., McGuire, L., Robles, T.F., et al. (2002b) Psychoneuroimmunology: psychological influences on immune function and health. *Journal of Consultative Clinical Psychology* 70: 537–547.

Kim, R.P., Edelman, S.V., Kim, D.D. (2001) Musculoskeletal complications of diabetes mellitus. *Clinical Diabetes* 19(3): 132–135.

Kimball, A.B., Yu, A.P., Signorovitch. J., et al. (2012) The effects of adalimumab treatment and psoriasis severity on self-reported work productivity and activity impairment for patients with moderate to severe psoriasis. *Journal of the American Academy of Dermatology* 66: e67–76.

Kimball, A.B., Gladman, D., Gelfand, J.M. (2008) National Psoriasis Foundation clinical consensus on psoriasis comorbidities and recommendations for screening. *Journal of American Academic Dermatology* 58: 1031–1042.

Kinzl, J.F., Traweger, C., Trefalt, E., et al. (2013) Psychosocial consequences of weight loss following gastric banding for morbid obesity. *Obesity Surgery* 13(1): 105–110.

Kircher, J.N., Park, M.H., Cheezum, M.K., et al. (2012) Cardiac tamponade in association with anorexia nervosa: a case report and review of the literature. *Cardiology Journal* 19: 635–638.

Klein, J.P. & Waxman, S.G. (2003) The brain in diabetes: molecular changes in neurons and their implications for end-organ damage. *Lancet Neurology* 2: 548–554.

Klok, M.D., Jakobsdottir, S., Drent, M.L. (2007) The role of leptin and ghrelin in the regulation of food intake and body weight in humans: a review. *Obesity Review* 8: 21–34.

Kofta, M., Weary, G., Sedek, G., et al. (1998) *The Emotional Control of Behavior. Personal Control in Action*: Springer, 133–154.

Kong, M-F. & Jevcoate, W. (1994) Eighty-six cases of Addison's disease. *Clinical Endocrinology* 41: 757–761.

Koronouri, O., Maguire, A.M., Knip, M., et al. (2009) Other complications and conditions associated with diabetes in children and adolescents. *Journal of Pediatric Diabetes.* 10(12): 204–210.

Koslow, S.H., Stokes, P.E., Mendels, J., et al. (1982) Insulin tolerance test: human growth hormone response and insulin resistance in primary unipolar depressed, bipolar depressed and control subjects. *Psycholicine* 12: 45–55.

Koubaa, S., Hallstrom, T., Lindholm, C. (2005) Pregnancy and neonatal outcomes in women with eating disorders. *Obstetrics* & Gynaecology 105: 255–260.

Kovacs, M., Ivengar, S., Goldston, D., et al. (1990) *Psychological functioning of children with insulin-dependent diabetes mellitus: a longitudinal study. Journal of Paediatric Psychology 15:* 619–632.

Kraeft, J.J., Uppot, R.N., Heffess, A.M. (2013) Imaging findings in eating disorders. *American Journal of Research/American Journal of Roentgenology* 200: W328–W335.

Kroenke, K., Jackson, J.L., Chamberlin, J. (1997) Depressive and anxiety disorders in patients presenting with physical complaints: clinical predictors and outcome. *American Journal of Medicine* 103(5): 339–347.

Kubik, J.F., Gill, R.S., Laffin, M., et al. (2013) The impact of bariatric surgery on psychological health. *Journal of Obesity.* http://dx.doi.org/10.1155/2013/837989

Kung, H.C., Hoyert, D.L., Xu, J.Q., et al. (2008) Deaths: final data for 2005. *National Vital Statistics Reports* 56(10) http://www.cdc.gov/nchs/data/nvsr/nvsr56/nvsr56_10.pdf

Kurd, S.K., Troxel, A.B., Crits-Christoph, P., et al. (2010) The risk of depression, anxiety, and suicidality in patients with psoriasis: a population-based cohort study. *Archive of Dermatology* 146: 891–895.

La Greca, A.M., Swales, T., Klemp, S., et al. (1995) Adolescents with diabetes: gender differences in psychosocial functioning and glycaemic control. *Children's Health Care* 24: 61–74.

Lai, Y., Wang, J., Jiang, F., et al. (2011) The relationship between serum thyrotropin and components of metabolic syndrome. *Endocrine Journal* 58(1): 23–30.

Laake, J.P., Stahl, D., Amiel, S.A., et al. (2014) The association between depressive symptoms and systemic inflammation in people with type 2 diabetes: findings from the South London Diabetes Study. *Diabetes Care* 37: 2186–2192.

Lampinen, P., Heikkinen, R-L., Ruoppila, I. (2000) Changes in intensity of physical exercise as predictors of depressive symptoms among older adults: an eight-year follow-up. *Preventative Medicine* 30(5): 371–380.

Larger, E. (2005) Weight gain & insulin treatment. *Diabetes Metabolism* 31: 4S51–4S56.

Lauret, E. & Rodrigo, L. (2013) Celiac disease and autoimmune-associated conditions. *Biomedical Research International.* http://gx.do1.org/10.1155/2013/127589.

Lavda, A.C., Webb, T.L., Thompson, A.R. (2012) A meta-analysis of the effectiveness of psychological interventions for adults with skin conditions. *British Journal of Dermatology* 167: 970–979.

Lazaro, L., Andres, S., Calvo, A., et al. (2013) Normal gray and white matter volume after weight restoration in adolescents with anorexia nervosa. *International Journal of Eating Disorders* 46: 481–488.

Ledhill, G., Rangel, L., Garralda, E. (2000) Surviving chronic physical illness, psychosocial outcome in adult life. *Archives of Disease in Childhood* 83: 104–110.

Leedom, L., Meehan, W.P., Procci, W., et al. (1991) Symptoms of depression in patients with type II diabetes mellitus. *Psychosomatics* 32: 280–286.

Leeds, J.S., Hopper, A.D., Hadjivassiliou, M., et al. (2011) High prevalence of microvascular complications in adults with type 1 diabetes and newly diagnosed celiac disease. *Diabetes Care* 34(10): 2158–2163.

Lehmer, L.M. & Ragsdale, B.D. (2012) Calcified periarthritis: more than a shoulder problem. *The Journal of Bone and Joint Surgery in America* 94(21): e157.

Leong, K.S., Wallymahmed, M., Wilding, J., et al. (1999) Clinical presentation of thyroid dysfunction and Addison's disease in young adults with type 1 diabetes. *Postgraduate Medical Journal* 75(886): 467–470.

Levenson, R.W. (1999) The Intrapersonal Functions of Emotion. *Cognition and Emotion* 13: 481–504.

Levin, R.J. & Smyth, D.H. (1963) The effect of the thyroid gland on intestinal absorption of hexoses. *The Journal of Physiology* 169: 755–769.

Leventhal, H., Benyamini, Y., Brownlee, S., et al. (1997) *Illness representations: theoretical foundations.* In: *Perceptions of Health and Illness*, Keith, J.P., John, W., (Eds.) Amsterdam: Harwood Academic, 155–188.

Levy, M.I. & Davis, K.L. (1983) The neuroendocrinology of depression. In: *Schizophrenia and Affective Disorders: Biology and Drug Treatment.* Rifkin, A. (Ed.), Boston: John Wright/PSG.

Ley, P. (1992) Improving patients' understanding, recall, satisfaction and compliance. In: *Health Psychology Process and Applications.* Broom, A. (Ed.) London: Chapman and Hall.

Ley, P. (1988) *Communicating With Patients: Improving Communication, Satisfaction, and Compliance.* New York: Croom Helm.

Lewis, M.D. (2005) Bridging emotion theory and neurobiology through dynamic systems modeling. *Behavioural Brain Science* 28: 169–194; discussion 194–245.

Lin, E.H., Von Korff, M., Katon, W., et al. (1995) The role of the primary care physician in patients' adherence to antidepressant therapy. *Medical Care* 33(1): 67–74.

Littlefield, C.H., Craven, J.L., Rodin, G.M., et al. (1992) Relationship of self-efficacy and bingeing to adherence to diabetes regimen among adolescents. *Diabetes Care* 15: 90–94.

Littell, J.H. & Girvin, H. (2002) Stages of Change: a critique'. *Behaviour Modification* 26(2): 22–27.

Litwak, L., Goh, S-Y., Hussein, Z., et al. (2013) Prevalence of diabetes complications in people with Type 2 diabetes mellitus and its association with baseline characteristics in the multinational $A_i$chive study. *Diabetology and Metabolic Syndrome* 5(57): http://www.dmsjournal.com/content/5/1/57

Litzelman, D.K., Slemenda, C.W., Langefeld, C.D., et al. (1993) Reduction of lower extremity clinical abnormalities in patients with non-insulin-dependent diabetes mellitus. A randomized, controlled trial. *Annals of Internal Medicine* 119: 36–41.

Lloyd, C., Smith, J., Weinger, K. (2005) Stress and Diabetes: A Review of the Links. *Diabetes Spectrum* 18: 121–127.

Locke, E.A. & Latham, G.P. (2002) Building a practically useful theory of goal setting and task motivation: a 5-year odyssey. *The American Psychologist* 57(9): 705–717.

Lok, C.F. & Bishop, G.D. (1999) Emotion control, stress, and health. *Psychology and Health* 14: 813–827.

Lo Sauro, C., Ravaldi, C., Cabras, P.L. (2008) Stress, hypothalamic-pituitary-adrenal axis and eating disorder. *Neuropsychobiology* 57: 95–115.

Lombardi, F., Franzese, A., Iafusco, D., et al. (2010) Bone involvement in clusters of autoimmune diseases: just a complication? *Bone* 46(2): 551–555.

Loveman, E., Frampton, G.K., Clegg, A.J. (2008) The clinical effectiveness of diabetes education models for Type 2 diabetes: a systematic review. *Health Technology Assessment* 12: 1–116, iii.

Löwe, B., Zipfel, S., Buchholz, C., et al. (2001) Long-term outcome of anorexia nervosa in a prospective 21-year follow-up study. *Psychology Medicine* 31: 881–890.

Lucas, S. & Walker, R. (2004) An overview of diabetes education in the United Kingdom: past, present and future. *Practical Diabetes International* 21: 61–64.

Ludvigsson, J.F., Elfstrom. P., Broom, U. (2007) Celiac disease and risk of liver disease: a general population-based study. *Clinical Gastroenterology and Hepatology* 5(1): 63–69.

Ludvigsson, J.F., Ludvigsson, J., Ekbom, A., et al. (2006) Celiac disease and risk of subsequent type 1 diabetes: a general population cohort study of children and adolescents. *Diabetes Care* 29(11): 2483–2488.

Lustman, P.J., Clouse, R.E., Nix, B.D., et al. (2006) Sertraline for prevention of depression recurrence in diabetes: a randomized, double-blind, placebo-controlled trial. *Archive of General Psychiatry* 63(5): 521–529.

Lustman, P.J., Clouse, R.E., Ciechanowski, P.S., et al. (2005) Depression-related hyperglycemia in type 1 diabetes: a mediational approach. *Psychosomatic Medicine* 67:195–199.

Lustman, P.J. & Clouse, R.E. (2002) Treatment of depression in diabetes: impact on mood and medical outcome. *Journal of Psychosomatic Research* 53: 917–924.

Lustman, P.J., Anderson, R.J., Freedland, K.E., et al. (2000a) Depression and poor glycaemic control: a meta-analytic review of the literature. *Diabetes Care* 23: 434–442.

Lustman, P.J., Freedland, K.E., Griffith, L.S., et al. (2000b) Fluoxetine for depression in diabetes: a randomized double-blind placebo controlled trial. *Diabetes Care* 23(5): 618–623.

Lustman, P.J., Clouse, R.E., Freedland, K.E. (1998a) Management of major depression in adults with depression: implications of recent clinical trials. *Seminars in Clinical Neuropsychiatry* 2: 15–23.

Lustman, P.J., Griffith, L.S., Freedland, K.E., et al. (1998b) Cognitive behavior therapy for depression in type 2 diabetes mellitus. A randomized, controlled trial. *Annuls of Internal Medicine* 129(8): 613–621.

Lustman, P.J., Clouse, R.E., Griffith, L.S., et al. (1997a) Screening for depression in diabetes using the Beck Depression Inventory. *Psychosomatic Medicine* 59: 24–31.

Lustman, P.J., Griffith, L.S., Freedland, K.E., et al. (1997b) The course of major depression in diabetes. *General Hospital Psychiatry* 19(2): 138–143.

Lustman, P.J., Griffith, L.S., Clouse, R.E., et al. (1997c) Effects of nortriptyline on depression and glycemic control in diabetes: results of a double-blind, placebo-controlled trial. *Psychosomatic Medicine* 59: 241–250.

Lustman, P.J., Griffith, L.S., Gavard, J.A., et al. (1992) Depression in adults with diabetes. *Diabetes Care* 15: 1631–1639.

Lustman, P.J., Carney, R.M., Clouse, R.E. (1988) Depression and the reporting of diabetes symptoms. *International Journal of Psychiatry Medicine* 18: 295–303.

Lustman, P.J. & Harper, G.W. (1987) Psychiatric physicians' identification and treatment of depression in patients with diabetes. *Comprehensive Psychiatry* 28: 22–27.

Lutfey, K.E. & Wishner, W.J. (1999) Beyond "compliance" is "adherence". Improving the prospect of diabetes care. *Diabetes Care* 22: 635–639.

Lyoo, I.K., Yoon, S., Jacobson, A.M., et al. (2012) Prefrontal cortical deficits in type 1 diabetes mellitus: brain correlates of comorbid depression. *Archives of General Psychiatry* 69: 1267–1276.

MacCuish, A.C. & Irvine, W.J (1975) Autoimmunological aspects of diabetes mellitus. *Clinical Endocrinology and Metabolism* 4: 435–471.

Maes, M., Lin, A.H., Delmeire, L., et al. (1999) Elevated serum interleukin-6 (IL-6) and IL-6 receptor concentrations in posttraumatic stress disorder following accidental man-made traumatic events. *Biology and Psychiatry* 45: 833–839.

Mafauzy, M. (2002) Repaglinide versus glibenclamide treatment of type 2 diabetes during Ramadan fasting. *Diabetes Research and Clinical Practice* 58: 45–53.

Mafauzy, M., Mohammed, W.B., Anum, M.Y., et al. (1990) A study of the fasting diabetic patient during the month of Ramadan. *Medical Journal of Malaysia* 45: 14–17.

Maggard, M.A., Shugarman, L.R., Suttorp, M., et al. (2005) Meta-analysis: surgical treatment of obesity. *Annals of Internal Medicine* 142(7): 547–559.

Mahmud, F.H., Murray, J.A., Kudva, Y.C., et al. (2005) Celiac disease in type 1 diabetes mellitus in a North American community: prevalence, serologic screening, and clinical features. *Mayo Clinic Proceedings* 80(11): 1429–1434.

Mainardi, E., Montanelli, A., Dotti, M., et al. (2002) Thyroid-related autoantibodies and celiac disease: a role for a gluten-free diet? *Journal of Clinical Gastroenterology* 35(3): 245–248.

Mainous, A.G., Tanner, R.J., Baker, R., et al. (2014) Prevalence of prediabetes in England from 2003 to 2011: population-based, cross-sectional study. *British Medical Journal* 4:e005002. doi: 10.1136/bmjopen-2014005002.

Mamplekou, E., Komesidou, V., Bissias, C., et al. (2005) Psychological condition and quality of life in patients with morbid obesity before and after surgical weight loss. *Obesity Surgery* 15(8): 1177–1184.

Mannucci, I., Rotella, F., Ricca, V., et al. (2005) Eating disorders in patients with Type 1 diabetes: a meta-analysis. *Journal of Endocrinological Investigation* 28: 417–419.

Marianna, R., Olga, B., Tzvi, B., et al. (2006) TH1/TH2 cytokine balance in patient with both type 1 diabetes mellitus and asthma. *Cytokine* 34:170–176.

Marinari, G.M., Papadia, F.S., Briatore, L. (2006) Type 2 diabetes and weight loss following biliopancreatic diversion for obesity. *Obesity Surgery* 16: 1440–1444.

Marliss, E.B. & Vranic, M. (2002) Insulin release and its role in glucoregulation: Implications for diabetes. *Diabetes* 51(1): S271–S283.

Markowitz, J.T., Butler, D.A., Volkening, L.K., et al. (2010) Brief screening tool for disordered eating in diabetes: internal consistency and external validity in a contemporary sample of pediatric patients with type 1 diabetes. *Diabetes Care* 33: 495–500.

Marks, V. & Richmond, C. (2007) *Insulin Murders: True Life Cases.* London: The Royal Society of Medicine Press Limited.

Marks, D.F., Murray, M., Evans, B., et al. (2000) *Health Psychology: Theory, Research and Practice.* London: Sage Publications.

Marple, R.L., Kroenke, K., Lucey, C.R., et al. (1997) Concerns and expectations in patients presenting with physical complaints: frequency, physician perceptions and actions, and 2-week outcome. *Archive of Internal Medicine* 157: 1482–1488.

Maratou, E., Hadjidakis, D.J., Kollias, A., et al. (2009) Studies of insulin resistance in patients with clinical and subclinical hypothyroidism. *European Journal of Endocrinology* 160(5): 785–790.

Maslow, A.H. (1943) A theory of human motivation. *Psychology Revisited* 50: 370.

Matty, A.J. & Seshadri, B. (1965) Effect of thyroxine on the isolated rat intestine. *Gut* 6: 200–202.

Maxon, H.R., Kreines, K.W., Goldsmith, R.E., et al. (1975) Long-term observations of glucose tolerance in thyrotoxic patients. *Archives of Internal Medicine* 135(11): 1477–1480.

Mayer-Davis, E.J., Sparks, K.C., Hirst, K., et al. (2004) Dietary intake in the diabetes prevention program cohort: baseline and 1-year post-randomisation. *Annals of Epidemiology* 14: 763–772.

Mazze, R., Lucido, D., Shampoon, H. (1984) Psychological and social correlates of glycaemic control. *Diabetes Care* 7: 360–366.

McAuley, E. & Blissmer, B. (2000) Self-efficacy determinants and consequences of physical activity. *Exercise & Sports Science Reviews* 28: 85–88.

McAuley, V. & Frier, B.M. (1999) Addison's disease in Type 1 diabetes presenting with recurrent hypoglycaemia. *Postgraduate Medicine* 76: 227–236.

McGill, J.B., Lustman, P.J., Griffith, L.S., et al. (1992) Relationship of depression to compliance with self-monitoring of blood glucose (Abstract). *Diabetes* 41: A84.

McKellar, J.D., Piette, J.D., Humphreys, K. (2004) Does self-care adherence mediate the relationship between depression and subsequent diabetes symptoms? *The Diabetes Educator* 30(3): 485–491.

McPherson, K., Marsh, T., Brown, M. (2007) *Foresight. Tackling Obesities: Future Choices – Modelling Future Trends in Obesity and the Impact on Health.* Second edition, London: government office for Science, Department of Innovation, universities and Skills.

Mc Sharry, J., Moss-Morris, R., Kendrick, T. (2011) Illness perceptions and glycaemic control in diabetes: a systematic review with meta-analysis. *Diabetic Medicine* 28: 1300–1310.

Melfi, C.A., Chawla, A.J., Croghan, T.W., et al. (1998) The effects of adherence to antidepressant treatment guidelines on relapse and recurrence of depression. *Archive of General Psychiatry.* 55(12): 1128–1132.

Mehler, P.S. & Brown, C. (2015) Anorexia nervosa – medical complications. *Journal of Eating Disorders* http://www.jeatdisord.com/content/3/1/11

Mehler, P.S., Sabel, A.L., Watson, T., et al. (2008) High risk of osteoporosis in male patients with eating disorders. *International Journal of Eating Disorders* 41: 666–672.

Mehta, N.N., Azfar, R.S., Shin, D.B., et al. (2010) Patients with severe psoriasis are at increased risk of cardiovascular mortality: cohort study using the General Practice Research Database. *European Heart Journal* 31: 1000–1006.

Meloni, A., Mandas, C., Jores, R.D., et al. (2009) Prevalence of autoimmune thyroiditis in children with celiac disease and effect of gluten withdrawal. *The Journal of Pediatrics*, 155(1): 51–55.

Mertens, V.C., Bosma, H., Groffen, D.A., et al. (2012) Good friends, high income or resilience? What matters most for elderly patients? *European Journal of Public Health* 22: 666–671.

Metso, S., Hyytia-Ilmonen, H., Kaukinen, K., et al. (2012) Gluten-free diet and autoimmune thyroiditis in patients with celiac disease. A prospective controlled study. *Scandinavian Journal of Gastroenterology* 47(1): 43–48.

Michie, S., Johnston, M., Abraham, C, et al., on behalf of the Psychological Theory group (2005). Making psychological theory useful for implementing evidence based practice: a consensus approach. *Quality and Safety in Health Care* 14: 26–33. www.psychol.ucl.

Miki, N., Ono, M., Hizuka, N., et al. (1992) Thyroid hormone modulation of the hypothalamic growth hormone (GH)-releasing factor-pituitary GH axis in the rat. *Journal of Clinical Investigation*, 90(1): 113–120.

Miller, K.K., Grinspoon, S.K., Ciampa, J. (2005) Medical findings in outpatients with anorexia nervosa. *Archive of Intern Medicine.* 165: 561–566.

Miller, W.R. & Rollnick, S. (2002) *Motivational Interviewing: Preparing People for Change*, Second edition. New York, London: The Guilford Press.

Mizara, A., Papadopoulos, L., McBride, S.R. (2012) Core beliefs and psychological distress in patients with psoriasis and atopic eczema attending secondary care: the role of schemas in chronic skin disease. *British Journal of Dermatology* 166: 986–993.

Misra, M. & Klibanski, A. (2014) Anorexia nervosa and bone. *Journal of Endocrinology* 221: R163-R176.

Misra, D.P., Das, S., Sahu, P.K. (2012) Prevalence of inflammatory markers (high-sensitivity C-reactive protein, nuclear factorκB, and adiponectin) in Indian patients with type 2 diabetes mellitus with and without macrovascular complications. *Metabolic Syndrome Related Disorder* 10: 209–213.

Moffitt, T.E., Arseneault, L., Belsky, D., et al. (2011) A gradient of childhood self-control predicts health, wealth, and public safety. *Proceedings of the National Academy of Scienc* 108: 2693-2698.

Mokuno, T., Uchimura, K., Hayashi, R., et al. (1999) Glucose transporter 2 concentrations in hyper- and hypothyroid rat livers. *Journal of Endocrinology* 160(2): 285–289.

Monnier, L., Colette, C., Owens, D.R. (2009) Integrating glycaemic variability in the glycaemic disorders of type 2 diabetes: a move towards a unified glucose tetrad concept. *Diabetes Metabolism Research and Review* 25: 393–402.

Monnier, L., Mas, E., Ginet, C., et al. (2006) Activation of oxidative stress by acute glucose fluctuations compared with sustained chronic hyperglycemia in patients with type 2 diabetes. *Journal of the American Medical Association* 295: 1681–1687.

Morris, L.G., Stephenson, K.E., Herring, S. (2004) Recurrent acute pancreatitis in anorexia and bulimia. *Journal of Physiology* 5: 231–234.

Morrisson, E.L. (2012) Diabetes and eating disorders – Together they're linked with a double dose of health consequences. *Today's Dietician* 14(12): 40–44.

Morton, I. & Hall, J.M. (1999) *Dictionary of Pharmacological Agents: Properties and Symptoms.* Springer Science & Business.

Moulik, P.K., Mtonga, R., Gill, G.V. (2003) Amputation and mortality in new-onset diabetic foot ulcers stratified by etiology. *Diabetes Care* 26(2): 491–494.

Mulrow, C.D. (2000) Case finding instruments for depression in primary care. *Annuls of Internal Medicine* 15: 123(12): 966.

Munday, H. (1996) Psychological aspects of diabetes care. *Diabetes Nursing* 23: 13–15.

Muraven, M., Gagné, M., Rosman, H. (2008) Helpful self-control: Autonomy support, vitality, and depletion. *Journal of Experimental Social Psychology* 44: 573–585.

Muraven, M., Baumeister, R.F., Tice, D.M. (1999) Longitudinal improvement of self-regulation through practice: building self-control strength through repeated exercise. *Journal of Social Psychology* 139: 446–457.

Murray, C.J.L. & Lopez, A.D. (1997) Global mortality, disability, and the contribution of risk factors: Global Burden of Disease Study. *Lancet* 349:1436–1442.

Murray, C.J.L. & Lopez, A.D. (1996) *The Global Burden of Disease: A Comprehensive Assessment of Mortality and Disability From Diseases, Injuries, and Risk Factors in 1990 and Projected to 2020.* Cambridge, Massachusetts: Harvard University Press.

Musselman, D.L., Betan, E., Larsen, H., et al. (2003) Relationship of depression to diabetes types 1 and 2: epidemiology, biology, and treatment. *Biological Psychiatry* 54: 317–329.

Myers, D.G. (2000) The funds, friends, and faith of happy people. *American Psychology* 55: 56–67.

Myers, E.D. & Branthwaite, A. (1992) Outpatient compliance with antidepressant medication. *British Journal of Psychiatry* 160: 83–86.

Myhre, A.G., Aarsetøy, H., Undlien, D.E., et al. (2013) High frequency of coeliac disease among patients with autoimmune adrenocortical failure. *Scandinavian Journal of Gastroenterology* 38(5): 511–515.

Naidoo, J. & Wills, J. (1994) *Health Promotion: Foundations for Practice.* London and Philadelphia: Balliere Tindall Limited.

Naka, K.K., Papathanassiou, K., Bechlioulis, A., et al. (2012) Determinants of vascular function in patients with type 2 diabetes. *Cardiovascular Diabetology* 11: 127.

Nalysnyk, L., Hernandez-Medina, M., Krishnarajah, G. (2010) Glycaemic variability and complications in patients with diabetes mellitus: evidence from a systematic review of the literature. *Diabetes, Obesity and Metabolism* 12: 288–298.

National Health Service (2000) *NHS Plan 2000*. London: Department of Health.

National Institute for Health and Care Excellence (NICE) (2014a) *The management of Type 2 diabetes*. London: NICE. nice.org.uk/cg87

National Institute for Health and Care Excellence (NICE) (2014b) Press release: NICE updates weight-loss surgery criteria for people with Type 2 diabetes. nice.org.uk/cg190

National Institute for Health and Care Excellence (NICE) (2014c) *Obesity identification assessment and management of overweight and obesity in children, young people and adults*. nice.org.uk/cg189

National Institute for Health and Clinical Excellence (NICE) (2004) *Eating Disorders. Core Interventions in the Treatment of and Management of Anorexia Nervosa, Bulimia Nervosa and Related Eating Disorders*. National Institute for Clinical Excellence, Clinical Guideline 9. http://guidance.nice.org.uk

National Institute for Health and Clinical Excellence (NICE) (2003) *Technical Appraisal Guidance No. 57: Guidance on the use of Continuous Subcutaneous Insulin Infusion for Diabetes*. London: NICE.

Niego, S.H., Kofman, M.D., Weiss, J.J., et al. (2007) Binge eating in the bariatric surgery population: a review of the literature. *International Journal of Eating Disorders* 40(4): 349–359.

Neimann, A.L., Shin, D.B., Wang, X., et al. (2006) Prevalence of cardiovascular risk factors in patients with psoriasis. *Journal of American Academic Dermatology* 55: 829-835.

Nielsen, S., Emborg, C., Molbak, A-G. (2002) Mortality in concurrent type 1 diabetes and anorexia nervosa. *Diabetes Care* 25:309–312.

Netzel, P.J., Mueller, P.S., Rummans, T.A., et al. (2002) Safety, efficacy, and effects on glycemic control of electroconvulsive therapy in insulin-requiring type 2 diabetic patients. *Journal of Electroconvulsive Therapy* 18: 16–21.

Neuhausen, S.L., Steele, S., Ryan, S., et al. (2008) Co-occurrence of celiac disease and other autoimmune diseases in celiacs and their first-degree relatives. *Journal of Autoimmunity* 31 (2): 160–165.

Neumark-Sztainer, D., Patterson, J., Mellin, A., et al. (2002) Weight control practices and disordered eating behaviours among adolescent females and males with Type 1 diabetes: associations with socio-demographics, weight concerns, familial factors and metabolic outcomes. *Diabetes Care* 25: 1289–1296.

Neumark-Sztainer, D., Story, M., Toporoff, F., et al. (1996) Psychosocial predictors of binge eating and purging behaviors among adolescents with and without diabetes mellitus. *Journal of Adolescent Healthcare* 19: 289–968.

Nerup, J. (1974) Addison's disease. Clinical studies: a report of 108 cases. *Acta Endocrinol* 76: 127–41.

Nuevo,R., Chatterji, S., Fraguas, D., et al. (2011) Increased risk of diabetes mellitus among persons with psychotic symptoms: Results from the WHO World Health Survey. *Journal of Clinical Psychiatry* 72: 1592–1599.

Newcomer, J.W. (2005) Second-generation (atypical) antipsychotics and metabolic effects: comprehensive literature review. *Central Nervous System Drugs* 19 (Supplement 1):1–93.

Nichols, G.A., Brown, J.B. (2003) Unadjusted and adjusted prevalence of diagnosed depression in type2 diabetes. *Diabetes Care* 26 (3): 744–749.

Nicolucci, A., Burns, K., Holt, R.I., et al. (2013) Diabetes Attitudes, Wishes and Needs second study (DAWN2): cross-national benchmarking of diabetes-related psychosocial outcomes for people with diabetes. *Diabetes Medicine* 30: 767–777.

Noar, S.M. & Zimmerman, R.S. (2005) Health Behavior Theory and cumulative knowledge regarding health behaviors: are we moving in the right direction? *Health Education Research* 20: 275–290.

O'Brien, J.P.E., Dixon, J.B., Laurie, C., et al. (2006) Treatment of mild to moderate obesity with laparoscopic adjustable gastric banding or an intensive medical program: a randomized trial. *Annals of Internal Medicine* 144(9): 625–633.

O'Leary, C., Walsh, C.H., Wieneke, P., et al. (2002) Coeliac disease and autoimmune Addison's disease: a clinical pitfall. *Monthly Journal of the Association of Physicians* 95(2): 79–82.

O'Leary, A., Shoor, S., Lorig, K., et al. (1988) A cognitive behavioural treatment for rheumatoid arthritis. *Health Psychology* 7: 527–542.

O'Meara, N.M., Blackman, J.D., Sturis, J., et al. (1993) Alterations in the kinetics of C-peptide and insulin secretion in hyperthyroidism. *Journal of Clinical Endocrinology and Metabolism* 76(1): 79–84.

Ouchi, N. & Walsh, K. (2007) Adiponectin as an anti-inflammatory factor. *Clinica Chima Acta* 380: 24–30.

Okamura, F., Tashiro, A., Utumi, A., et al. (2000) Insulin resistance in patients with depression and its changes during the clinical course of depression: minimal model analysis. *Metabolism and Clinical Experiment* 49: 1255–1260.

Okajima, F. & Ui, M. (1979) Metabolism of glucose in hyper- and hypothyroid rats in vivo. Glucose-turnover values and futilecycle activities obtained with 14C- and 3H-labelled glucose. *Biochemical Journal* 182(2): 565–575.

Oyibo, S.O., Jude, E.B., Tarawneh, I., et al. (2001) The effects of ulcer size and site, patient's age, sex and type and duration of diabetes on the outcome of diabetic foot ulcers. *Diabetes Medicine* 18(2): 133–138.

Palinkas, L.A., Barrett-Connor, E., Wingard, D.L. (1991) Type 2 diabetes and depressive symptoms in older adults: a population-based study. *Diabetic Medicine* 8: 532–539.

Panksepp, J. (2007) Neurologizing the psychology of Affects: How appraisal-based constructivism and basic emotion theory can coexist. *Perspectives on Psychological Science* 2: 281–296.

Park, M., Katon, W.J., Wolf, F.M. (2013) Depression and risk of mortality in individuals with diabetes: a meta-analysis and systematic review. *General Hospital Psychiatry* 35: 217–225.

Patarca, R., Klimas, N.G., Lugtendorf, S., et al. (1994) Dysregulated expression of tumor necrosis factor in chronic fatigue syndrome: interrelations with cellular sources and patterns of soluble immune mediator expression. *Clinical Infectious Disease* 18(Supplement 1): S147–S153.

Pavy, F.W. (1885) Introductory address to the discussion of the clinical aspects of glycosuria. *Lancet* 2: 1085–1087.

Penckofer, S., Quinn, L., Byrn, M., et al. (2012) Does glycemic variability impact mood and quality of life? *Diabetes and Technological Therapy* 14: 303–310.

Penninx, B.W., Kritchevsky, S.B., Yaffe, K., et al. (2003) Inflammatory markers and depressed mood in older persons: results from the Health, Aging and Body Composition study. *Biology and Psychiatry* 54: 566–572.

Penno, G., Solini, A., Bonora, E., et al. (2013) HbA1c variability as an independent correlate of nephropathy, but not retinopathy, in patients with type 2 diabetes: the Renal Insufficiency And Cardiovascular Events (RIACE) Italian multicenter study. *Diabetes Care* 36: 2301–2310.

Petty, R., Sensky, T., Mahler, R. (1991) Diabetologists' assessments of their outpatients' emotional state and health beliefs: accuracy and possible sources of bias. *Psychotherapy and Psychosomatics* 55(2-4):164–169.

Peveler, R.C., Bryden, K.S., Neil, A.W., et al. (2005) The relationship of disordered eating habits and attitudes to clinical outcomes in young adult females with type 1 diabetes. *Diabetes Care* 28(1): 84–88.

Peveler, R.C., Carson, A., Rodin, G. (2002) Depression in medical patients. *British Medical Journal* 325: 149–152.

Peveler, R.C., Fairburn, C.G., Boller, I., et al. (1992) Eating disorders in adolescents with IDDM: a controlled study. *Diabetes Care* 15:1356–1360.

Peraira, R.F. & Alvarenga, M. (2007) Disordered eating: identifying, treating, preventing, and differentiating it from eating disorders. *Diabetes Spectrum* 20(3): 140–146.

Pessoa, L. (2008) On the relationship between emotion and cognition. *National Review of Neuroscience* 9: 148–158.

Peyrot, M. & Rubin, R.R. (2007) Behaviour and psychosocial interventions in diabetes. *Diabetes Care* 2433–2440.

Peyrot, M. & Rubin, R.R. (1997) Levels and risks of depression and anxiety symptomology among diabetic adults. *Diabetes Care* 20: 585–590.

Pham-Short, A., Donaghue, K.C., Ambler, G., et al. (2010) Coeliac disease in type 1 diabetes from 1990 to 2009: higher incidence in young children after longer diabetes duration. *Diabetic Medicine* 29(9): e.286–e.289.

Phelps, E.A. (2006) Emotion and cognition: insights from studies of the human amygdala. *Annual Review of Psychology* 57: 27–53.

Picot, J., Jones, J., Colquitt, J.L., et al. (2009) The clinical effectiveness and cost-effectiveness of bariatric (weight loss) surgery for obesity: a systematic review and economic evaluation. *Health Technology Assessment* 13(41): 1–190, 215–357.

Piette, J.D., Richardson, C., Valenstein, M. (2004) Addressing the needs of patients with multiple chronic illness: the case of diabetes and depression. *The American Journal of Managed Care* 10(2): 152–164.

Piette, J.D., Schillinger, D., Potter, M.B., et al. (2003) Dimensions of patient-provider communication and diabetes self-care in an ethnically-diverse population. *Journal of General Internal Medicine* 18: 1–10.

Podnos, Y.D., Jimenez, J.C., Wilson, S.E., et al. (2003) Complications after laparoscopic gastric bypass: a review of 3464 cases. *Archives of Surgery* 138: 957– 961.

Pollock, M., Kovacs, M., Chartron-Prochownik, D. (1995) Eating disorders and mal-adaptive dietary/insulin management among youths with childhood-onset insulin-dependent diabetes mellitus. *Journal of the American Academy of Child and Adolescent Psychiatry* 34: 291–296.

Polli, N., Blengino, S., Moro, M., et al. (2006) Pericardial effusion requiring pericardiocentesis in a girl with anorexia nervosa. *International Journal of Eating Disorders* 39: 609–611.

Pop-Bisui, R. (2010) Cardiac autonomic neuropathy in diabetes. *Diabetes Care* 33(2): 434–441.

Porcelli, P., Leandro, G., De Carne, M. (1998) Functional gastrointestinal disorders and eating disorders. Relevance of the association in clinical management. *Scandinavian Journal of Gastroenterology* 33: 577–582.

Pories, W.J., Swanson, M.S., MacDonald, K.G., et al. (1995) Who would have thought it? An operation proves to be the most effective therapy for adult-onset diabetes mellitus. *Annuls of Surgery* 222: 339–350; discussion 350–352.

Pound, N., Chipchase, S., Treece, K., et al. (2005) Ulcer-free survival following management of foot ulcers in diabetes. *Diabetes Medicine* 22(10): 1306–1309.

Pouwer, F., Beekman, A.T., Nijpels, G., et al. (2003) Rates and risks for co-morbid depression in patients with type 2 diabetes mellitus: results from a community-based study. *Diabetologia.* 46(7): 892–898.

Pouwer, F., Snoek, F.J., van der, Ploeg, H.M., et al. (2001) Monitoring of psychological well-being in patients with diabetes: Effects on mood, HbA1c and the patient's evaluation of the quality of diabetes care: a randomised controlled trial. *Diabetes Care* 24: 1929–1935.

Preskorn, S.H. (2000) The adverse effect of the profiles of the selective serotonin reuptake inhibitor's relationship to invitro pharmaceuticals. *Journal of Psychological Practice* 6(3): 151–154.

Prime, N. (1987) *Introduction to Pathology for Radiographers.* London: Harper and Row Limited.

Prochaska, J.O., Velicer, W.F. (1997a) The Transtheoretical model of health behaviour change. *American Journal of Health Promotion* 12: 38–48.

Prochaska, J.O. & Velicer, W.F. (1997b) Misinterpretation and misapplication of the Transtheoretical model. *American Journal of Health Promotion* 12: 11–12.

Prochaska, J.O. (1992) What causes people to change from unhealthy to health-enhancing behaviour? In: *Preventing Cancers,* Heller, T., Bailey, L., and Pattison, S. (Eds.) Milton Keynes: Open University Press.

Prochaska, J.P. & DiClemente, C.C. (1984) *The Transtheoretical Approach: Crossing Traditional Boundaries of Change.* Illinois: Don Jones/Irwin Homewood.

Radloff, L.S. (1977) The CES-D Scale: a self-report depression scale for research in the general population. *Applied Psychological Measurement* 1: 385–401.

Ramasubbu, R. (2002) Insulin resistance: a metabolic link between depressive disorder and atherosclerotic vascular diseases. *Medical Hypotheses* 59: 537–551.

Ramacciotti, C.E., Coli, E., Biadi, O. (2003) Silent pericardial effusion in a sample of anorexic patients. *Eating and Weight Disorders* 8: 68–71.

Rane, K., Wajngot, A., Wändell, P.E., et al. (2011) Psychosocial problems in patients with newly diagnosed diabetes: number and characteristics. *Diabetes Research and Clinical Practice* 93: 371–378.

Reiter, J., Wexler, I.D., Shehadeh, N., et al. (2007) Type 1 diabetes and prolonged fasting. *Diabetic Medicine* 24: 436–439.

Rendell, M. (2004) The role of sulphonylureas in the management of type 2 diabetes mellitus. *Drugs* 64: 1339–1358.

Retnakaran, R. & Zinman, B. (2009) Thiazolidinediones and clinical outcomes in type 2 diabetes. *Lancet* 373: 2088–2090.

Reunala, T., Salmi, J., Karvonen, J. (1987) Dermatitis herpetiformis and celiac disease associated with Addison's disease. *Archives of Dermatology* 123(7): 930–932.

Revicki, D.A., Menter, A., Feldman, S., et al. (2008) Adalimumab improves health-related quality of life in patients with moderate to severe plaque psoriasis compared with the United States general population norms: results from a randomized, controlled Phase III study. *Health Quality and Life Outcomes* 6: 75.

Rezek, M. (1976) The role of insulin in the glucostatic control of food intake. *Canadian Journal of Physiology and Pharmacology* 54: 650–665.

Rezzonico, J., Rezzonico, M., Pusio, E.l., et al. (2008) Introducing the thyroid gland as another victim of the insulin resistance syndrome. *Thyroid* 18(4): 461–464.

Rich, L.M., Caine, M.R., Findling, J.W. (1990) Hypoglycemic coma in anorexia nervosa. Case report and review of the literature. *Archive of Intern Medicine* 150: 894–895.

Robertson, S.M., Amspoker, A.B., Cully, J.A., et al. (2013) Affective symptoms and change in diabetes self-efficacy and glycaemic control. *Diabetes Medicine* 30: e189–e196.

Robertson, S.M., Stanley, M.A., Cully, J.A., et al. (2012) Positive emotional health and diabetes care: concepts, measurement, and clinical implications. *Psychosomatics* 53: 1–12.

Robbins, L.B., Pender, N.J., Ronis, D.L., et al. (2004) Physical activity, self-efficacy and perceived exertion among adolescents. *Research in Nursing & Health* 27: 435–446.

Rochon, C., Tauveron, I., Dejax, C., et al. (2003) Response of glucose disposal to hyperinsulinaemia in human hypothyroidism and hyperthyroidism. *Clinical Science* 104(1): 7–15.

Rodin, G., Olmsted, M.P., Rydall, A.C., et al. (2002) Eating behaviour in obese patients with and without Type 2 diabetes mellitus. *International Journal of Obesity-Related Metabolic Disorders* 26: 848–853.

Rollnick, S., Mason, P., Butler, C. (2000) *Health Behavior Change: A Guide for Practitioners.* Churchill Livingstone: London.

Rossi, S.R., Greene, G.W., Reed, G., et al. (1997) Diabetes self-management: self-report of the recommendations, rates and patterns in a large population. *Diabetes Care* 4: 568–576.

Rossi, S.R., Greene, G.W., Reed, G., et al. (1994a) Continuous investigation of a process of change measure for dietary fat reduction. *American Behavioural Medicine* 16 (Supplement): 167.

Rossi, S.R., Greene, G.W., Reed, G., et al. (1994b) Cross-validation of a decisional balance measure for dietary fat reduction. *American Behavioural Medicine* 16 (Supplement): 167.

Rothwell, P.M., Howard, S.C., Dolan, E., et al. (2010) Prognostic significance of visit-to-visit variability, maximum systolic blood pressure,
and episodic hypertension. *Lancet* 375: 895–905.

Rubiano, F., Kaplan, L.M., Schauer, P.R., et al. (2010a) Diabetes Surgery
Summit Delegates. The Diabetes Surgery Summit consensus conference: recommendations for the evaluation and use of gastrointestinal
surgery to treat type 2 diabetes mellitus. *Annuls of Surgery* 251: 399–
405.

Rubiano, F., Forgione, A., Cummings, D.E., et al. (2006a) The mechanism
of diabetes control after gastrointestinal bypass surgery reveals a role
of the proximal small intestine in the pathophysiology of type 2 diabetes. *Annuls of Surgery* 244: 741–749.

Rubiano, F. (2006b) Bariatric surgery: effects on glucose homeostasis.
Current Opinion in Clinical Nutrition and Metabolic Care 9: 497–507.

Ruggiero, L. (2000) Helping people with diabetes change behaviour: from
theory to practice. *Diabetes Spectrum* 13: 125–137.

Ruggiero, L. & Prochaska, J.O. (1993) Readiness to change: application of
the Transtheoretical model to diabetes. *Diabetes Spectrum* 6(1): 22–24.

Rush, M.R., Whitebird, R.R., Rush, M.R., et al. (2008) Depression in patients with diabetes: Does it impact clinical goals? *Journal of the
American Board of Family Medicine* 21(5): 392–397.

Russell, R.C. (2012) *Diabetic Ketoacidosis.* Seattle, Washington: VSD Publications.

Rutter, M. (2013) Annual Research Review: Resilience--clinical implications. *Journal of Child Psychology and Psychiatry* 54: 474–487.

Rutter, M. (2012) Resilience as a dynamic concept. *Developmental Psychopathology* 24: 335–344.

Rutter, M. (2006) Implications of resilience concepts for scientific understanding. *Annals of the New York Academy of Science* 1094: 1–12.

Rydall, A.C., Rodin, G.M., Olmsted, M.P., et al. (1997) Disordered eating behavior and microvascular complications in young women with
insulin-dependent diabetes mellitus. *New England Journal of Medicine* 336:1849–1854.

Ryff, C.D., Dienberg Love, G., et al. (2006) Psychological well-being and ill-being: do they have distinct or mirrored biological correlates? *Psychotherapy and Psychosomatics* 75: 85–95.

Sabel, A.L., Rosen, E., Mehler, P. (2014) Severe anorexia nervosa in males: clinical presentations and medical treatment. *Eating Disorders* 22: 209–220.

Sabel, A.L., Gaudiani, J.L., Statland, B. (2013) Hematological abnormalities in severe anorexia nervosa. *Annals of Hematology* 92: 605–613.

Sainsbury, A., Sanders, D.S., Ford, A.C. (2011) Meta-analysis: coeliac disease and hypertransaminasaemia. *Alimentary Pharmacology and Therapeutics* 34(1): 33–40.

Salardi, S., Volta, U., Zucchini, S., et al. (2008) Prevalence of celiac disease in children with type 1 diabetes mellitus increased in the mid-1990s: an 18-year longitudinal study based on antiendomysial antibodies. *Journal of Pediatric Gastroenterology and Nutrition* 46(5): 612–614.

Sanchez-Zaldıvar, S., Arias-Horcajadas, F., Gorgojo-Martınez, J.J., et al. (2009) Evolution of psychopathological alterations in patients with morbid obesity after bariatric surgery. *Medicina Clininca* 33(6): 206–212.

Sarwer, D.B., Dilks, R.J., Ritter, S. (2012) *Bariatric Surgery for Weight Loss: Encyclopedia of Body Image and Human Appearance*, vol. 1. San Diego, California: Academic Press.

Sarwar, N., Gao, P., Seshasai, S.R., et al. (2010) Diabetes mellitus, fasting blood glucose concentration, and risk of vascular disease: a collaborative meta-analysis of 102 prospective studies. *Lancet* 375: 2215–2222.

Sategna-Guidetti, C., Volta, U., Ciacci, C., et al. (2001) Prevalence of thyroid disorders in untreated adult celiac disease patients and effect of gluten withdrawal: an Italian multicenter study. *American Journal of Gastroenterology* 96(3): 751–757.

Saydah, S.H., Brancati, F.L., Golden, S.H., et al. (2003) Depressive symptoms and the risk of type 2 diabetes mellitus in a US sample. *Diabetes Metabolic Research Revised* 19(3): 202–208.

Schauer, P.R., Burguera, B., Ikramuddin, S., et al. (2003) Effect of laparo-scopic Roux-en Y gastric bypass on type 2 diabetes mellitus. *Annuls of Surgery* 238: 467–484; discussion 84–85.

Scheff, T.J. (1983) Toward integration in the social psychology of emotions. *Annual Review of Sociology* 9: 333–354.

Schernthaner, G., Grimaldi, A., Di Mario, U. (2004) GUIDE study: double-blind comparison of once-daily gliclazide MR and glimepiride in type 2 diabetic patients. *European Journal of Clinical Investigation* 34: 535–542.

Schernthaner, G. & Morton, J.M. (2008) Bariatric surgery in patients with morbid obesity and type 2 diabetes. *Diabetes Care* 31(2): S297–S302,

Schleifer, J., Macari-Hinson, M.M., Coyle, D.A., et al. (1989) The nature and course of depression following myocardial infarction. *Archives of Internal Medicine* 149(8): 1785–1789.

Schulberg, H.C., Katon, W.J., Simon, G.E., et al. (1999) Best clinical practice: guidelines for managing major depression in primary medical care. *Journal of Clinical Psychiatry* 60 (supplement 7): 19–26.

Schwartz, S.A., Weissberg-Benchell, J., Perlmuter, L.C. (2000) Personal control and disordered eating in female adolescents with type 1 diabetes. *Diabetes Care* 25: 1987–1991.

Schwarzer, R. & Fuchs, R. (1995) Self-efficacy & health behaviours. In: *Predicting Health Behaviour & Practice with Social Cognition Models.* Buckingham: Open University Press.

Schweiger, C., Weiss, R., Keidar, A. (2010) Effect of different bariatric operations on food tolerance and quality of eating. *Obesity Surgery* 20: 1393–1399.

Schwimmer, J.B., Burwinkle, T.M., Varni, V.W. (2003) Health-related quality of life of severely obese children and adolescents. *Journal of the American Medical Association* 289(14): 1813–1819.

Scopinaro, N., Marinari, G., Camerini, G., et al. (2005) 2004 ABS Consensus Conference: Biliopancreatic diversion for obesity: state of the art. *Surgery and Obesity* 1: 317–328.

Segerstrom, S.C. & Miller, G.E. (2004) Psychological stress and the human immune system: a meta-analytic study of 30 years of inquiry. *Psychology Bulletin* 130: 601–630.

Seligman, M.E. (1975) *Helplessness.*San Francisco: Freeman.

Sestoft, L., Christensen, N.J., Saltin, B. (1991) Responses of glucose and glucoregulatory hormones to exercise in thyrotoxic and myxoedematous patients before and after 3 months of treatment. *Clinical Science* 81(1): 91–99.

Shaban, C. (2013) Diabulimia: mental health condition or media hyperbole? *Practical Diabetes* 30(3): 104–105a.

Shai, I., Henkin, Y., Weitzman, S., et al. (2003) Determinants of long-term satisfaction after vertical banded gastroplasty. *Obesity Surgery* 13(2): 269–274.

Shaw, K.M. & Cummings, M.H. (2005) *Diabetes: Chronic Complications.* Second edition, Chichester: John Wiley and Sons Limited.

Sheldon, K.M., Williams, G., Joiner, T. (2000) *Self Determination Theory in the Clinic: Motivating Physical and Mental Health.* New Haven: Yale University Press.

Shibata, S., Saeki, H., Tada, Y. (2009) Serum high molecular weight adiponectin levels are decreased in psoriasis patients. *Journal of Dermatological Science* 55: 62–63.

Shilitoe, R.W. (1988) *Psychology and Diabetes: Psychological Factors in Management and Control.* London: Chapman and Hall.

Shikiar, R., Heffernan, M., Langley, R.G., et al. (2007) Adalimumab treatment is associated with improvement in health-related quality of life in psoriasis: patient-reported outcomes from a phase II randomized controlled trial. *Journal of Dermatology and Treatment* 18: 25–31.

Simon, G.E. & Von Korff, M. (1995) Recognition, management, and outcomes of depression in primary care. *Archive of Family Medicine* 4(2): 99–105.

Simsek, D.G., Aycan, S., Ozen, Z., et al. (2013) Diabetes care, glycemic control, complications, and concomitant autoimmune diseases in children with type 1 diabetes in Turkey: a multicenter study. *Journal of Clinical Research in Pediatric Endocrinology* 22(5): 20–26.

Sindrup, S.H., Ejlertsen, B., Gjessing, H., et al. (1988) Peripheral nerve function during hyperglycaemic clamping in healthy subjects. *Acta Neurolgica Scandinavia* 78:141–145.

Singer, M.A. (2001) Of mice and men and elephants: metabolic rate sets glomerular filtration rate. *American Journal of Kidney Diseases* 37(1): 164–178.

Singh, N.A., Clements, K.M., Singh, M.A. (2001) The efficacy of exercise as a long-term antidepressant in elderly subjects: a randomized, controlled trial. *Journal of Gerontology, Biological Science and Medical Science* 56(8): M497–504.

Sinha, S., Munichoodappa, C.S., Kozak, G.P. (1972) Neuroarthropathy in diabetes mellitus. *Medicine* 51: 191–210.

Sirey, J.A., Bruce, M.L., Aplexopoulos, G.S., et al. (2001a) Stigma as a barrier to recovery: perceived stigma & patient-related severity of illness as predictors of anti-depressant drug adherence. *Psychiatric Services* 52(12): 1615–1620.

Sirey, J., Bruce, M.L., Raue, P., et al. (2001b) Psychological barriers in young and older outpatients with depression as predictors of treatment discontinuation. *American Journal of Psychiatry* 158: 479–481.

Skaff, M.M., Mullan, J.T., Almeida, D.M., et al. (2009) Daily negative mood affects fasting glucose in type 2 diabetes. *Health Psychology* 28: 265–272.

Sjöström, C.D., Lissner, L., Wedel, H., et al. (1999) Reduction in incidence of diabetes, hypertension and lipid disturbances after intentional weight loss induced by bariatric surgery: the SOS intervention study. *Obesity Research* 7(5): 477–484.

Sjöström, L., Lindroos, A.K., Peltonen, M., et al. (2004) Swedish Obese Subjects Study Scientific Group. Lifestyle, diabetes, and cardiovascular risk factors 10 years after bariatric surgery. *New England Journal of Medicine* 351: 2683–2693.

Skinner, T.C., Carey, M.E., Cradock, S., et al. (2010) Depressive symptoms in the first year from diagnosis of Type 2 diabetes: results from the DESMOND trial. *Diabetes Medicine* 27: 965–967.

Skroubis, G., Sakellaropoulos, G., Pouggouras, K., et al. (2002) Comparison of nutritional deficiencies after Roux-en-Y gastric bypass and after biliopancreatic diversion with Roux-en-Y gastric bypass. *Obesity Surgery* 12: 551– 558.

Slevin, E. (2004) High intensity counselling or behavioural interventions can result in moderate weight loss. *Evidence-based Healthcare* 8: 16–18.

Smith, R.W., Korenblum, C., Thacker, K. (2013) Severely elevated transaminases in an adolescent male with anorexia nervosa. *International Journal of Eating Disorders* 46: 751–754.

Smyth, J.M. & Arigo, D. (2009) Recent evidence supports emotion regulation interventions for improving health in at-risk and clinical populations. *Current Opinion in Psychiatry* 22: 205–210.

Sniehotta, F.F., Scholz, U., Schwarzer, R. (2005) Bridging the intention-behaviours gap: planning, self-efficacy, and action control in the adoption and maintenance of physical exercise'. *Psychology and Health* 20(2): 14–60.

Snow, V., Lascher, S., Mottur-Pilson, C. (2000) Pharmacologic treatment of acute major depression and dysthymia. *Annuls of Internal Medicine* 132(9): 738–742.

Sola, E., Morillas, C., Garzon, S., et al. (2002) Association between diabetic ketoacidosis and thyrotoxicosis. *Acta Diabetologica* 39(4): 235–237.

Sollid, L.M., Qiao, S-W., Anderson, R.P., et al. (2012) Nomenclature and listing of celiac disease relevant gluten T-cell epitopes restricted by HLA-DQ molecules. *Immunogenetics* 64 (6): 455–460.

Sommerfield, A.J., Deary, I.J., Frier, B.M. (2004) Acute hyperglycaemia alters mood state and impairs cognitive performance in people with Type 2 diabetes. *Diabetes Care* 27: 2335–2340.

Songar, A., Kocabasoglu, N., Balcioglu, I., et al. (1993) The relationship between diabetics' metabolic control levels and psychiatric symptomatology. *Integrated Psychiatry* 9: 34–40.

Spadaccino, A.C., Basso, D., Chiarelli, S., et al. (2008) Celiac disease in North Italian patients with autoimmune thyroid diseases. *Autoimmunity* 41(1): 116–121.

Spaner, D., Bland, R.C., Newman, S.C. (1994) Epidemiology of psychiatric disorders in Edmonton: major depressive disorder. *Acta Psychiatry Scandinavian Supplement* 376: 7–15.

Spelman, L.M., Walsh, P.I., Sharifi, N., et al. (2007) Impaired glucose tolerance in first-episode drug-naïve patients with schizophrenia. *Diabetic Medicine* 24: 481–485.

Sowunmi, A. (1993) Psychosis after cerebral malaria in children. *Journal of the National Medical Association* 85: 695–696.

Sponzilli, I., Chiari, G., Iovane, B., et al. (2010) Celiac disease in children with type 1 diabetes: impact of gluten free diet on diabetes management. *Acta Biomedica* 81(3): 165–170.

Stagi, S., Giani, T., Simonini, G., et al. (2005) Thyroid function, autoimmune thyroiditis and coeliac disease in juvenile idiopathic arthritis. *Rheumatology* 44 (4): 517–520.

Stanford Patient Education Research Center (2012) Program Fidelity Manual: Stanford Self-Management Programs 2012 Update. Stanford University.

http://patienteducation.stanford.edu/licensing/FidelityManual2012.pdf

Starkey, K. & Wade, T. (2010) Disordered eating in girls with Type 1 diabetes: examining directions for prevention. *Clinical Psychologist* 14(1): 2–9.

Steel, J.M., Young, R.J., Lloyd, G.G., et al. (1987) Clinically apparent eating disorders in young diabetic women: associations with painful neuropathy and other complications. *British Medical Journal* 294: 859–862.

Steenkamp, D., Patel, V., Minkin, R. (2011) A case of pneumomediastinum: a rare complication of diabetes. *Clinical Diabetes* 29(2): 76–77.

Steinhardt, M.A., Mamerow, M.M., Brown, S.A., et al. (2009) A resilience intervention in African American adults with type 2 diabetes: a pilot study of efficacy. *Diabetes Educator* 35: 274–284.

Sterry, W., Strober, B.E., Menter, A. (2007) Obesity in psoriasis: the metabolic, clinical and therapeutic implications. Report of an interdisciplinary conference and review. *British Journal of Dermatology* 157: 649–655.

Stone, J.B., Bluhm, H.P., White, M.I. (1984) Correlates of depression among long-term insulin-dependent diabetics. *Rehabilitation Psychology* 29: 85–93.

Stratton, I.M., Adler, A.I., Neil, H.A., et al. (2000) Association of glycaemia with macrovascular and microvascular complications of type 2 diabetes (UKPDS 35): prospective observational study. *British Medical Journal* 21: 405–412.

Strumia, R. (2005) Dermatologic signs in patients with eating disorders. *American Journal of Clinical Dermatology* 6: 1-10.

Stuckey, H.L., Mullan-Jensen, C.B., Reach, G., et al. (2014) Personal accounts of the negative and adaptive psychosocial experiences of people with diabetes in the second Diabetes Attitudes, Wishes and Needs (DAWN2) study. *Diabetes Care* 37: 2466–2474.

Stunkard, A.J. & Wadden, T.A. (1992) Psychological aspects of severe obesity. *American Journal of Clinical Nutrition* 55(2): 524S–532S.

Sullivan, M.D., Katon, W.J., Lovato, L.C., et al. (2013) Association of depression with accelerated cognitive decline among patients with type 2 diabetes in the ACCORD-MIND trial. *Journal of the American Medical Association of Psychiatry* 70: 1041–1047.

Sun, J.K., Keenan, H.A., Cavallarano, J.D., et al, (2011) Protection from retinopathy and other complications in patients with Type 1 diabetes of extreme duration. *Diabetes Care* 34: 968–974.

Svenson, M., Engström, I., Aman, J., et al. (2003) Higher drive for thinness in adolescent males with insulin-dependent diabetes mellitus compared with healthy controls. *Acta Paediatrica* 12: 122–128.

Taguchi, S., Oinuma, T., Yamada, T. (2000) A comparative study of cultured smooth muscle cell proliferation and injury, utilizing glycated low density lipoproteins with slight oxidation, auto-oxidation, or extensive oxidation. *Journal of Atherosclerosis and Thrombosis* 7: 132–137.

Takahashi, H., Tsuji, H., Takahashi, I., et al. (2008) Plasma adiponectin and leptin levels in Japanese patients with psoriasis. *British Journal of Dermatology* 159: 1207–1208.

Takki, M., Uchigata, Y., Nozzaki, A.T., et al. (2002) Classification of Type 1 diabetic females with bulimia nervosa into sub-groups according to purging behaviour. *Diabetes Care* 25(9): 1664–1665.

Talbot, F. & Nouwen, A. (2000) A review of the relationship between depression and diabetes in adults: is there a link? *Diabetes Care* 23: 1556–1562.

Tam, L.S., Tomlinson, B., Chu, T.T., et al. (2008) Cardiovascular risk profile of patients with psoriatic arthritis compared to controls--the role of inflammation. *Rheumatology* 47: 718–23.

Tamer, E., Gur, G., Polat, M., et al. (2009) Flare-up of pustular psoriasis with fluoxetine: possibility of a serotoninergic influence? *Journal of Dermatology Treatment* 20: 137–140.

Tan Pei Lin, L. & Kwek, S.K. (2010) Onset of psoriasis during therapy with fluoxetine. *General Hospital Psychiatry* 32: 446: e9–10.

Taylor, S.E. (1995) *Health Psychology*. London: McGraw-Hill.

Tew, J.D. Jr., Mulsant, B.H., Haskett, R.F., et al. (1999) Acute efficacy of ECT in the treatment of major depression in the old. *American Journal of Psychiatry* 156: 1865–1870.

The Eurodiab Ace Study Group and the Eurodiab Ace Substudy 2 Study Group (1998) Familial risk of type I diabetes in European children. *Diabetologia* 41: 1151–1156.

Thoolen, B.J., de Ridder, D., Bensing, J., et al. (2009) Beyond good intentions: The role of proactive coping in achieving sustained behavioural change in the context of diabetes management. *Psychology and Health* 24: 237–254.

Tiberti, C., Panimolle, P., Bonamico, M., et al. (2012) IgA antitransglutaminase autoantibodies at type 1 diabetes onset are less frequent in adult patients and are associated with a general celiac-specific lower immune response in comparison with nondiabetic celiac patients at diagnosis. *Diabetes Care* 35(10): 2083–2085.

Tice, D.M., Baumeister, R.F., Shmueli, D., et al. (2007) Restoring the self: Positive affect helps improve self-regulation following ego depletion. *Journal of Experimental Social Psychology* 43: 379–384.

Tiemens, B.G., Von Korff, M., Lin, E.H.B. (1998) Diagnosis of depression by primary care physicians versus a structured diagnostic interview. *General Hospital Psychiatry* 21(2): 87–96.

Tiemens, B.G., Ormel, J., Simon, G.E. (1996) Occurrence, recognition, and outcome of psychological disorders in primary care. *General Hospital Psychiatry* 153(5): 636–644.

Timonen, M., Laakso, M., Jokelainen, J., et al. (2005) Insulin resistance and depression: cross-sectional study. *British Medical Journal* 330:17–18, 2005

Tobin, A.M., Veale, D.J., Fitzgerald, O., et al. (2010) Cardiovascular disease and risk factors in patients with psoriasis and psoriatic arthritis. *Journal of Rheumatology* 37:1386–1394.

Tones, K. & Tilford, S. (1994) *Health Education: Effectiveness, Efficiency and Equity,* Second edition, London: Chapman & Hall. 92: 114-117.

Tortora, G.J. & Grabowski, S.R. (1993) *Principles of Anatomy and Physiology.* Seventh edition, New York: Harper Collins.

Tosi, F., Moghetti, P., Castello, R., et al. (1996) Early changes in plasma glucagon and growth hormone response to oral glucose in experimental hyperthyroidism. *Metabolism* 45(8): 1029–1033.

Triolo, T.M., Armstrong, T.K., McFann, K., et al. (2011) Additional autoimmune disease found in 33% of patients at type 1 diabetes onset. *Diabetes Care* 34 (5): 1211–1213.

Tsai, A.G. & Wadden, T.A. (2005) Systematic review: an evaluation of major commercial weight loss programs in the United States. *Annuls of Intern Medicine* 142: 56–66.

Tseng, C.L., Soroka, O., Maney, M. (2014) Assessing potential glycemic overtreatment in persons at hypoglycemic risk. *Journal of the American Medical Association Internal Medicine* 174: 259–268.

Tsukayama, E., Toomey, S.L., Faith, M.S., et al. (2010) Self-control as a protective factor against overweight status in the transition from childhood to adolescence. *Archive of Pediatric and Adolescent Medicine* 164: 631–635.

Tyring, S., Gottlieb, A., Papp, K., et al. (2006) Etanercept and clinical outcomes, fatigue, and depression in psoriasis: double-blind placebo-controlled randomized phase III trial. *Lancet* 367: 29–35.

UKPDS Group (1998a) Intensive blood glucose control with sulfonylureas or insulin compared with conventional treatment and risk of complications in patients with type 2 diabetes (UKPDS 33). *Lancet* 352: 837–853.

UKPDS Group (1998b) Effect of intensive blood glucose control with metformin on complications in overweight patients with type 2 diabetes (UKPDS 34). *Lancet* 352: 854–865.

Ulger, Z., Gürses, D., Ozyurek, A.R. (2006) Follow-up of cardiac abnormalities in female adolescents with anorexia nervosa after refeeding. *Acta Cardiology* 61: 43–49.

Utiger, R.D. (1995) Altered thyroid function in nonthyroidal illness and surgery. To treat or not to treat? *New England Journal of Medicine* 7: 1562–1563.

Uysal, A.R., Erdogan, M.F., Sahin, G., et al. (1998) Clinical and metabolic effects of fasting in 41 type 2 diabetic patients during Ramadan (Letter). *Diabetes Care* 21: 2033–2034.

Vaccarino, V., Kasl, S.V., Abramson, J., et al. (2001) Depressive symptoms and risk of functional decline and death in patients with heart failure. *Journal of American Collective Cardiology* 38: 199-205.

Valerio, G., Spadaro, R., Iafusco, D., et al. (2008) The influence of gluten free diet on quantitative ultrasound of proximal phalanxes in children and adolescents with type 1 diabetes mellitus and celiac disease. *Bone* 43(2): 322-326.

Van Hout, G.C.M., Boekestein, P., Fortuin, F.A.M., et al. (2006) Psychosocial functioning following bariatric surgery. *Obesity Surgery* 16(6): 787-794.

Van Hout, G.C.M. (2005) Psychosocial effects of bariatric surgery. *Acta Chirurgica Belgica* 105(1): 40-43.

Vajro, P., Paolella, G., Maggiore, G., et al. (2003) Meta-analysis: pediatric celiac disease, cryptogenic hypertransaminasemia, and autoimmune hepatitis. *Journal of Pediatric Gastroenterology and Nutrition* 56(6): 663-670.

Van der Does, F.E., De Neeling, J.N., Snoek, F.J. (1996) Symptoms and well-being in relation to glycemic control in type II diabetes. *Diabetes Care* 19: 204-210.

Van de Laar, F.A., Lucassen, P.L., Akkermans, R.P., et al. (2005) Alpha-glucosidase inhibitors for type 2 diabetes mellitus. *Cochrane Database Systematic Review* CD003639.

Vander Wal, J.S. & Mitchell, E.R. (2011) Psychological complications of pediatric obesity. *Clinics of North America* 58(6): 1393-1401.

Vaughan, M. (1967) An in vitro effect of triiodothyronine on rat adipose tissue. *Journal of Clinical Investigation* 46(9): 1482-1491.

Vaxilliare, M. & Froguel, P. (2010) The genetics of Type 2 diabetes from candidate gene biology to genome-wide studies. In: Holt, R.I.G., et al. (Eds.) *Textbook of Diabetes.* Oxford: Wiley-Blackwell.

Ventura, A., Neri, E., Ughi, C., et al. (2000) Gluten-dependent diabetes-related and thyroid-related autoantibodies in patients with celiac disease. *The Journal of Pediatrics* 137(2): 263-265.

Verhoeven, E.W., Kraaimaat, F.W., de Jong, E.M., et al. (2009a) Effect of daily stressors on psoriasis: a prospective study. *Journal of Investigation into Dermatology* 129: 2075–2077.

Verhoeven, E.W., Kraaimaat, F.W., de Jong, E.M., et al. (2009b) Individual differences in the effect of daily stressors on psoriasis: a prospective study. *British Journal of Dermatology* 161: 295–299.

Vernon MC, Mavropoulos J, Transue M, et al. (2003) Clinical experience of a carbohydrate-restricted diet: Effect on diabetes mellitus. *Metabolic Syndrome and Related Disorders* 1: 233–238.

Viljamada, M., Kaukinen, K., Huhtala, H., et al. (2005) Coeliac disease, autoimmune diseases and gluten exposure. *Scandinavian Journal of Gastroenterology* 40 (4): 437–443.

Vileikyte, L., Leventhal, H., Gonzalez, J., et al. (2005) Diabetic peripheral neuropathy and depressive symptoms. *Diabetes Care* 28: 2378–2383.

Vohs, K.D., Glass, B.D., Maddox, W.T., et al. (2011) Ego depletion is not just fatigue: Evidence from a total sleep deprivation experiment. *Social Psychology and Personal Science* 2: 166–173.

Vohs, K.D. & Faber, R.J. (2007) Spent resources: Self-regulatory resource availability affects impulse buying. *Journal of Consumer Research* 33: 537–547.

Volta, U., de Franceschi, F., Lari, L., et al. (1998) Coeliac disease hidden by cryptogenic hypertransaminasaemia. *Lancet* 352(912): 26– 29.

Wahl. O. (1999) Mental health consumers' experience of stigma. *Schizophrenia Bulletin* 25: 467–478.

Wakkee, M., Thio, H.B., Prens, E.P., et al. (2007) Unfavorable cardiovascular risk profiles in untreated and treated psoriasis patients. *Atherosclerosis* 190: 1–9.

Walker, R.J., Smalls, B.L., Hernandez-Tejada, M.A., et al. (2012) Effect of diabetes fatalism on medication adherence and self-care behaviors in adults with diabetes. *General Hospital Psychiatry* 34: 598–603.

Walker, J.D., Young, R.J., Little, J., et al. (2002) Mortality in concurrent Type 1 diabetes and anorexia nervosa. *Diabetes Care* 25(9): 1571–1575.

Walter, R.E., Beiser, A., Givelber, R.J., et al. (2003) Association between glycemic state and lung function: the Framingham Heart Study. *American Journal of Respiration and Critical Care Medicine* 167: 911–916.

Wanless, D., Appleby, J., Harrison, A., et al. (2007). *Our Future Health Secured? A review of NHS funding and performance.* London: King's Fund.

Wang, Y., Chen, J., Zhao, Y., et al. (2008) Psoriasis is associated with increased levels of serum leptin. *British Journal of Dermatology* 158: 1134–1135.

Waterston, J. (1995) "Funny, you don't look like a diabetic". Bath: Ashgrove Press.

Wax, R. (2013) *Sane New World: Taming The Mind.* Croydon: Hodder & Stoughton.

Webb, T.L. & Sheeran, P. (2006) Does changing behavioural intentions engender behavioural change? A meta-analysis of the experimental evidence. *Psychological Bulletin* 12(20): 249–268.

Webb, T.L. & Sheeran, P. (2003) Can implementation intentions help to overcome ego-depletion? *Journal of Experimental and Social Psychology* 39: 279–286.

Weiden, P., Olfson, M., Essock, S. (1997) Medication noncompliance in schizophrenia: effects on mental health service policy. In: *Treatment Compliance and the Therapeutic Alliance: Chronic Mental Illness*, volume 5. Blackwell, B. (Ed.), Singapore: Harwood Academic.

Weinger, K., Jacobson, A.M., Draelos, M.T., et al. (1995) Blood glucose estimation and symptoms during hyperglycemia and hypoglycemia in patients with insulin-dependent diabetes mellitus. *American Journal of Medicine* 98: 22–31.

Weinman, J. & Petrie, K.J. (1997) Illness perceptions: a new paradigm for psychosomatics? *Journal of Psychosomatic Research* 42: 113–116.

Weiss, S.C., Kimball, A.B., Liewehr, D.J., et al. (2002) Quantifying the harmful effect of psoriasis on health-related quality of life. *Journal of American Academic Dermatology* 47: 512–518.

Weissman, M.M., Bland, R.C., Canino, G.J., et al. (1996) Cross-national epidemiology of major depression and bipolar disorder. *Journal of the American Medical Association* 276: 293–299.

West, R. (2006) *Theory of Addiction*. Oxford: Blackwell Publishing.

West, R. (2005) Time for a change: putting the transtheoretical (stages of change) model to rest. *Addiction* 100: 106–109.

Westman, E.C., Yancy, W.S., Mavropoulos, J.C., et al. (2008) The effect of a low-carbohydrate, ketogenic diet versus a low glycaemic index diet on glycaemic control in Type 2 diabetes mellits. *Nutrition and Metabolism* 5: 36.

Whitlock, G., Lewington, S., Sherliker, P., et al. (2009) Body-mass index and cause-specific mortality in 900,000 adults: collaborative analyses of 57 prospective studies. *Lancet* 373 (9669): 1083–1096.

Willey, K.A. & Singh, M.A. (2003) Battling insulin resistance in elderly obese people with type 2 diabetes: bring on the heavy weights. *Diabetes Care* 26:1580–1588.

Williams, J.W., Kerber, C.A., Mulrow, C.D., et al. (1995) Depressive disorders in primary care: prevalence, functional disability, and identification. *Journal of General Internal Medicine* 10(1): 7–12.

Williams, M.W., Clouse, R.E., Lustman, P.J. (2006) Understanding depression as a medical risk factor to prevent diabetes and its complications. *Clinical Diabetes* 24(2): 79–89.

Willis, T. (1971) *Diabetes: A Medical Odyssey*. New York: Tuckahoe.

Wilson, V.L. (2014) *Insulin: Uses and Abuses*. New York: Teneo Press.

Wilson, V.L. (2013) Type 2 diabetes in children and adolescents: a growing epidemic. *Nursing Children and Young People* 25(2): 14–17.

Wilson, V.L. (2009) Behavioural change in type 1 diabetes self-management: why and how? *Health Education Journal* 68(4): 320–327.

Wilson, V.L. (2007) Perceived support needs for intensive diabetes self-management. *Journal of Diabetes Nursing* 11(1): 8–13.

Wilson, V.L. (2005) Insulin Pump Therapy. In: *Structured Patient Education in Diabetes: Report from the Patient Education Working Group.* London: Department of Health/Diabetes UK.

Wilson, V.L. (2004a) Gastroparesis: a patient's experience. *Journal of Diabetes Nursing* 8(2): 73-75.

Wilson, V.L. (2004b) The NSF for Diabetes: addressing psychosocial issues. *Journal of Diabetes Nursing* 8(10): 372-376.

Wilson, V.L. (2003a) Survey of information and support needs of people with type 1 diabetes. *Journal of Diabetes Nursing* 7(7): 272–277.

Wilson, V.L. (2003b) Insulin pump therapy: the patient's perspective. *Diabetes and Primary Care* 5(3): 132–136.

Winokur, A., Maislin, G., Phillips, J.L. (1988) Insulin resistance after oral glucose tolerance testing in patients with major depression. *American Journal of Psychiatry* 145: 325–330.

Wooley, S.C. & Garner, D.M. (1991) Obesity treatment: the high cost of false hope. *Journal of the American Dietetic Association* 91(10): 1248–1251.

World Health Organisation (2011) *Diabetes.* Factsheet no: 312. Geneva: World Health Organisation.

World Health Organization (2000) *Obesity: Preventing and Managing the Global Epidemic. Report of a WHO Convention,* WHO Technical Report Series 894. Geneva: World Health Organization.

Worthy, D.A., Byrne, K.A., Fields, S. (2014) Effects of emotion on prospection during decision-making. *Frontiers of Psychology* 5: 591. doi: 10.3389/fpsyg.2014.00591

Yang, G.R., Yang, J.K., Zhang, L., et al. (2010) Association between subclinical hypothyroidism and proliferative diabetic retinopathy in type 2 diabetic patients: a case-control study. *Tokyo Journal of Experimental Medicine* 222(4): 303–310.

Yashuhara, D., Deguchi, D., Tsutsui, J. (2003) Reactive hypoglycemia induced by rapid change in eating behavior in anorexia nervosa. *International Journal of Eating Disorders* 34: 273–277

Yi, J.P., Vitaliano, P.P., Smith, R.E., et al. (2008) The role of resilience on psychological adjustment and physical health in patients with diabetes. *British Journal of Health Psychology* 13: 311–325.

Yi-Frazier, J.P., Smith, R.E., Vitaliano, P.P., et al. (2010) A person-focused analysis of resilience resources and coping in diabetes patients. *Stress and Health* 26: 51–60.

Yipp, I., Go, V.L., De Shields, S., et al. (2001) Lipid meal replacement and glycaemic control in obese Type 2 diabetes patients. *Obesity Research* 9(4): 341S–347S.

Young, E.A., Haskett, R.F., Murphy-Weinberg, V., et al. (1991) Loss of glucocorticoid fast feedback in depression. *Achieve of General Psychiatry* 48: 693–699.

Young, V., Eiser, C., Johnson, B., et al. (2013) Eating problems in adolescents with type 1 diabetes: a systematic review with meta-analysis. *Diabetes Medicine* 30: 189–198.

Young-Hyman, D.L. & Davis, C.L. (2010) *Disordered Eating in Individuals with Diabetes: Importance of Context, Evaluation and Classification.* American Diabetes Association http://creativecommons.org/licenses/by-nc-nd/3.0/

Yung-Tsung, H., Wen-Chien, C., Wei-Chih, L., et al. (2015) Type 1 diabetes and increased risk of subsequent asthma: a nationwide population-based cohort study. *Medicine* 94(36): pe1466.

Yusuf, S., Hawken, S., Ounpuu, S., et al. (2004) Effect of potentially modifiable risk factors associated with myocardial infarction in 52 countries (the INTERHEART study): case control study. *Lancet* 364: 937–952.

Zelissen, P.M., Bast, E.J., Croughs, R.J. (1995) Associated autoimmunity in Addison's disease. *Journal of Autoimmunity* 8: 121–130.

Zeller, M.H., Reiter-Purtill, J., Ratcliff, M.B., et al. (2011) Two-year trends in psychosocial functioning after adolescent Roux-en-Y gastric bypass. *Surgery for Obesity and Related Diseases* 7(6): 727–732.

Zeller, M.H., Roehrig, H.R., Modi, A.C., et al. (2006) Health-related quality of life and depressive symptoms in adolescents with extreme obesity presenting for bariatric surgery. *Pediatrics* 117, (4): 1155–1161.

Ziegelstein, R.C., Fauerbach, J.A., Stevens, S.S., et al. (2000) Patients with depression are less likely to follow recommendations to reduce cardiac risk during recovery from a myocardial infarction. *Archive of Internal Medicine* 160(12):1818–1823.

Index